Stabbed in the **BACK**

NORTIN M. HADLER, M.D.

Stabbed in the
BACK

CONFRONTING

BACK PAIN IN AN

OVERTREATED

SOCIETY

THE UNIVERSITY OF NORTH CAROLINA PRESS **CHAPEL HILL**

Designed by Courtney Leigh Baker and set
in Whitman and URW Grotesk by Rebecca Evans
Manufactured in the United States of America

The paper in this book meets the guidelines for permanence
and durability of the Committee on Production Guidelines
for Book Longevity of the Council on Library Resources.

The University of North Carolina Press has been a member
of the Green Press Initiative since 2003.

Library of Congress Cataloging-in-Publication Data
Hadler, Nortin M.
Stabbed in the back : confronting back pain in an
overtreated society / Nortin M. Hadler.
    p. cm.
Includes bibliographical references and index.
ISBN 978-0-8078-3348-3 (cloth : alk. paper)
1. Backache—Popular works. I. Title.
RD771.B217H33 2009
617.5′64—dc22
2009019737

CLOTH   13 12 11 10 09   5 4 3 2 1

A LIFETIME IN MEDICINE IS A RARE PRIVILEGE. *I am trusted to bring to the bedside the highest of intentions and a most highly informed understanding of the limits of certainty. For the degree that I am* **physician***, I owe much to mentors, colleagues, patients, and students. I have aspired to repay each in devotion and gratitude. The degree to which I am a complete physician results from the support, understanding, nurturing, and love of my wife, Carol. We have walked through life, hand in hand, for nearly forty-five years.*

CONTENTS

FIGURES AND TABLES

Figures

Tables

PREFACE

Studying and understanding the clinical, social, and policy implications of low back pain have occupied most of my research efforts for over thirty years. I joined the faculty of the University of North Carolina (UNC) in 1973; this was my first job after all the years of training. I was an eager clinician, educator, and investigator trained to pursue the causes of arthritis at a very basic scientific level.

Off I went to my first rheumatology clinic, proudly displaying a name tag that read "Assistant Professor of Medicine" and confident I knew all that was known about rheumatoid arthritis, lupus, scleroderma, and the other systemic diseases that are the purview of the academic rheumatologist. My first patient was a well-muscled man of forty, who appeared anxious and in some discomfort.

"Doc," he said, "I injured my back and I don't know if I can go to work."

If the complaint was, "My back has been getting stiffer and stiffer since I was a teenager," I would have been able to help him with his ankylosing spondylitis. But I had no experience or body of information to draw upon to help him with any component of his complaint—the pain in his back, the notion that his back was injured even though he couldn't point to a particular event or accident that had caused the injury, or the perception that he was too incapacitated as a result of his back pain to continue pursuing gainful employment. I examined him, reassured him that he had suffered no major structural catastrophe, and admitted that I knew not what else to do or say. I suggested that since he had been coping for a couple of months already, he should continue to do so, and I would see him in two weeks, prepared to offer him wiser counsel.

Those were an interesting two weeks. I read extensively; the literature on backache was copious but almost entirely an exercise in anecdote, preconception, and guesswork. I spoke with colleagues and was offered the same. Several senior colleagues advised me not to waste my time on this patient's disorder: "You're too good a physical biochemist to worry about such a nonacademic topic," they said. I dismissed that advice and commenced the intellectual odyssey that has resulted in this book.

Some of the chapters that follow are state-of-the-science discussions of aspects of this patient's initial complaint. Others are state-of-the-art discussions of aspects for which the science has proved no match. And still others are discussions of the context in which both the science and the art play out—the social, historical, political, and psychological contexts that transform the predicament of low back pain into an illness, even an incapacitating illness if not a disabling injury. The pathobiology of the spine accounts for the pain in the back; it is the context that causes the suffering.

That realization occurred early on, during that initial two weeks when I was shaking all the trees and hoping that some dollop of wisdom would fall out. If I was to understand the experience of the illness of backache, I would have to forge well beyond the science I had trained to study. For that I was prepared—much to my surprise at the time, but not in retrospect. Yes, I understood the scientific method and was comfortable with its empirical demands. But I also understood that the care of the patient was not an exercise in molecular biology. It still isn't and never will be.

I came of academic age when the model was the "three-legged stool": teaching, research, and administration. The last I have managed to avoid throughout my career, but "teaching" clinical medicine, to my way of thinking, demanded clinical expertise. Teaching and clinical expertise drive me to this day. I have listened to the plight of thousands of patients and learned to listen closely. No one suffers illness in a vacuum. No illness illustrates that aphorism better than regional backache. I was prepared to understand that, and willing to pursue its ramifications, from the moment I went to the bedside of that first patient who said, "Doc, I injured my back and I don't know if I can go to work."

Thirty-five years later, I know how to respond to such a plaint. By the time you finish reading *Stabbed in the Back*, you will know how to as well.

ACKNOWLEDGMENTS

David Perry is the editor in chief of the University of North Carolina Press. David Perry is also my colleague and has become my friend. He shepherded *Worried Sick* through the publishing gauntlet and has done as well by *Stabbed in the Back*. In doing so, he taught this physician-author how to be an author-physician. I am so grateful for his efforts on behalf of my work.

I am also grateful for the opportunity to work with the community of professionals that is the UNC Press. Dino Battista, Gina Mahalek, and Laura Gribbin are responsible for the public face of the book and Jay Mazzocchi for the high polish on its prose.

Stabbed in the **BACK**

INTRODUCTION

To live a year without a backache is abnormal.

Backache is an intermittent predicament of life. No one is spared for long. Furthermore, no approach to avoiding the next episode has proved effective when submitted to scientific testing. To be well is not to avoid backache; it is to have the wherewithal to cope with it effectively and repeatedly.

Almost all of the people we will be talking about in this book were afflicted with regional backache, and that is the only type of backache we will consider here. I coined that term for an editorial in the *New England Journal of Medicine* over twenty years ago.[1] Regional backache is the back pain experienced by people who are otherwise well. It comes on inexplicably, usually suddenly, in the course of activities that are familiar and customarily comfortable. This is the common, everyday backache. We will spend some time considering some of the more frequent complications of a regional backache, particularly the "pinched nerve," which can cause pain to radiate down the leg. We are not going to consider the unusual causes of backache, such as metastatic cancer, infections, or inflammatory diseases of the spine. Nor will we consider the back pain that can result from accidents and other traumatic events.

While I am talking about what this book is not, let me say that it is not a self-help manual. Nor is it a medical textbook. *Stabbed in the Back* is an exposé of a contrived "disease" and the enormous enterprises it has spawned that conspire to its "cure" and provide fallback when a "cure" is elusive. That industry has developed a life of its own despite a robust and compelling body of scientific investigation that points toward backache as a socially constructed ailment. The American notion of health, the

American's wherewithal to cope and persevere, and the American pocket-book are paying a heavy price.

An assault on the backache industry is long overdue. No reader will find all of the chapters that follow resting easily within his or her pre-conceptions. Many will find some of the information presented here to be counterintuitive, some of it infuriating. After all, no one has escaped backache; we all know someone who suffered mightily and probably some-one whose life is burdened with a "bad back." I am not out to rub salt in the wounds of sufferers. But I know no other way to help those yet to fall victim, and perhaps some who already have, than to forcefully and directly decry the status quo and to support my assertions with the science that society has ignored.

Clinical aspects of regional low back pain and the various treatments are discussed in the central chapters. My intent is to illustrate the fashion in which the state of the science could and should inform the state of the art. There are many relevant, reproducible, quantifiable scientific assertions about back pain. Some of the science leads to assertions that are counter-intuitive. Many are a reproach to "common practice." All are difficult to implement given the common wisdom about backache. Changing attitudes and entrenched practices is never quick and easy. I have written this book in the hope of greasing that path.

Over the ages, almost every causal and therapeutic notion imaginable, and some unimaginable, has been foisted on the individual who seeks assistance in coping with a regional backache. Furthermore, often, even more often than not, the assistance coincides with relief of the pain. Few who sought a "cure" would then regard the "cure" as a coincidence. Few who are "cured" can entertain the possibility that they were fooled, that they would have done as well without the "cure." Hence, "cures" become entrenched and over time succor their purveyors and their advocates, who are certain that their record of success is incontrovertible evidence that their diagnosis of the cause of the pain was valid and the "cure" worked. On the next flare-up of back pain, the firm believer is likely to return for another ministration. And if the result is less satisfactory, he is likely to as-sume that this episode of back pain is worse or different from the last and that another type of treatment needs to be superimposed. In this fashion, society convinces so many people that therapists hold the solution to their current or next backache. Testing all these parallel and intertwined, yet firmly held, beliefs is an enormous scientific challenge.

One of the greatest yet unsung accomplishments of the scientific method is to have largely met this challenge. In the past twenty years, not only have many of the theories regarding the avoidance of back pain been tested, but many of the proposed treatments have been systematically studied as well. None survives "unscathed," and most have been proven untenable. Each of the central chapters of this book examines a particular establishment committed to and succored by the present system: the physician, the alternative provider, and the surgeon. To the extent that each rests on untested beliefs, or beliefs that defy testing on methodological grounds, they are sectarian communities of providers. Many who are treated and most doing the treating balk at submitting their treatments to scientific testing. They fall back on metaphysical arguments, and they have the power and money to influence the polity and the common sense. All I can do is hope that this book will arm readers with the critical wherewithal to fend for themselves in this marketplace. I realize that the lag between the time that our preconceptions are formed and the time that we need to exercise informed choice can be many decades. All I can hope is that reason will prevail over sectarian interests and metaphysical arguments . . . someday.

In writing this book, I have several goals that relate to health-care policy. I have just stated the first. The second relates to the notion that a regional backache is an injury. The latter chapters in the book take on this idea. Prior to the 1940s, one would have been no more comfortable labeling a regional backache an "injury" than one would a headache. This change is not simply an exercise in labeling; it is an example of a linguistic determinism that accompanied the rise of a movement for a safer workplace.

Before the mid-twentieth century, almost no American worker had health insurance other than what was covered by workers' compensation schemes for an injury that occurred at work. The injured worker is indemnified for medical care and salary maintenance. It is not surprising that a hernia in the groin area would soon be labeled a "rupture" qualifying as a compensable injury. Backache soon followed. I can explain these roots in empathic terms. However, labeling regional back pain an injury has not afforded much advantage to the worker with regional low back pain. To the contrary, it has provided the workforce with relentless grief and the establishment committed to its perpetuation with unconscionable largesse. The phrase "I injured my back at work" and workers' compensation indemnity schemes go hand in hand. In the past two decades, the relationship has been carefully and scientifically explored, and the results are clear.

The final chapters of *Stabbed in the Back* dissect the ergonomic fallacy, the primacy of the context of work over the content of tasks, and our fatally flawed approach to disability determination. Again, my hope is that reason will prevail over the vast establishment vested in the status quo so that someday the plight of the worker with a back "injury" will evoke empathic treatment and not approaches that predispose to persistent suffering and disability. That will not happen until we all understand why a particular worker might find a predicament of normal life, a regional backache, to be disabling. These chapters, more than any others, are a product of my own research over the past thirty years.[2]

I have written extensively on the contemporary notion of "well-being"[3] and the fashion in which that social construction promotes the provision of irrational health care.[4] Today's backache is an object lesson. The implications for health-care reform are also clear and compelling.

Science has not arrived at contemporary understandings in a particularly straightforward fashion. Hypotheses are never generated in a vacuum; they always carry the baggage of what came before. The more powerful stakeholders somehow find a way to impose their views and preconceptions. Research into back pain is a case in point. And back-pain research is finally emerging into the light of reproducible results.

Metaphorically, one might imagine several enterprises vying to tunnel through a mountain of preconceptions about backache. Each stakes out a unique starting point. Their progress is determined by the amount of backing they have, and their paths are rendered erratic by false starts and unforeseen impediments. Each has its own sponsor with distinctive goals regarding prevention, causation, and treatment. Seldom do they share secrets. In fact, seldom do they take cognizance of each other as more than distant rumblings in adjacent passageways. Each excavation is leaving a mountain of detritus—the detritus of discarded hypotheses—at their tunnel entrance. This book compares and contrasts these tunnels to a degree that seldom occupies the excavators themselves. Most of these tunneling enterprises are now breaking through the crust of the other side of the mountain. The reader of *Stabbed in the Back* will be among the first to realize that all of them have come to a common egress.

ONE

Three Marks of the Past on
the Backs of the Present

Suffering low back pain today is quite different from suffering backache in past generations. Today's back pain is not your grandfather's lumbago. No doubt the pain is the same. No doubt the likelihood of experiencing the pain is the same. But the degree to which one suffers, the fashion in which one copes, one's notions of what caused the pain, and the menu of potential treatments are not the same. This variability over time and among people bears witness to the uncertainties regarding the cause and "cure" of low back pain.

Low back pain is not unique in this. Medieval societies found all sorts of explanations for the Black Death, from scapegoats to the metaphysical. Today no such thinking is a match for our understanding of the biology of the bacterium *Pasteurella pestis* and its passage from animals to humans. Medicine's inventiveness in the treatment of phthisis (consumption), even when we knew it to be pulmonary tuberculosis, seemed boundless. Light therapy for the disease garnered a Nobel Prize, rest cures were universally applied, and some surgical interventions seem bizarre in retrospect. All this vanished shortly after Selman Waksman discovered streptomycin, thereby garnering a Nobel Prize for a really effective treatment.

Low back pain has at least as colorful a history. Furthermore, since we still have no earthly idea what causes regional low back pain, new chapters in this history continue to be written today. Thanks to compelling scientific analysis, we do have a robust understanding of the clinical, social, and policy ramifications of the experience. Some of the notions held up as truth by past generations are more than colorful, however; some seem to have developed a life of their own despite science to the contrary; and some have an ancient history.

Sciatica

In Genesis 32:26, Jacob wrestles with a "man" who is generally interpreted to be an angel: "When he [the angel] perceived that he could not overcome him [Jacob], he struck [or wrenched] the socket of his hip; so Jacob's hip-socket was strained as he wrestled with him." A few verses later, in Genesis 32:32–33, "the sun rose for him [Jacob] as he passed Penuel [face of God] and he was limping on his hip." Jacob carries on, presumably healing nicely as there is no further mention of his limping. In both the Hebrew and King James versions, the major nerves of the thigh were held to be the source of Jacob's limping. Modern translations are more specific, impugning the sciatic nerve. For millennia, pains in the hip region and abnormalities of local neural structures have been intertwined. The Greek word for "hip," *ischion*, is the common root for the name of the bone-bearing the hip socket (ischium), the French word for "hip" (*hanche*), and sciatica.*

The ancients also endowed us with other notions of the cause of low back pain. Imhotep, the legendary and prolific physician to the Pharaoh around 2800 BCE, also left his mark as astrologer and priest and as the architect and engineer who served as general contractor for the construction of one of the step pyramids. Imhotep took advantage of the latter experience to observe and document the injuries to the workers involved in such

---

*If Jacob's experience left a mark, it is on the Jewish tradition if not the study of gross anatomy. "Therefore the Children of Israel are not to eat the displaced sinew [thigh muscle] on the hip-socket to this day, because he [the angel] struck Jacob's hip-socket on the displaced sinew." What structure is this "sinew"? The Hebrew *gid Ha-nashe* translates with difficulty. The King James Bible translates it as "sinew of the thigh"; other classic versions prefer "hollow of the thigh." Regardless of the translation, the major nerves of the thigh were long held to be the source of Jacob's limping. Modern translations impugn the sciatic nerve specifically. For example, *Les éditions du Cerf* and Bayard's *la bible* both translate Jacob's affliction: "Il a touché le creux de la hanche de Jacob, le nerf sciatique." To this day, the Orthodox Jewish tradition mandates that every last trace of the sciatic nerve, the common peroneal nerve, and nearly every other major nerve and vein coursing through an animal's hindquarter be removed ("traboring") before the meat is deemed kosher and fit for human consumption. This stipulation, detailed by the Sages of the Talmud (Chullin 91a), is based on the passages in Genesis, not the dietary laws that were written later and codified in Leviticus 11 and Deuteronomy 14.

a dangerous and physically demanding endeavor. Low back pain is afforded detailed treatment in his writings.[1]

In a scroll known as the Edwin Smith Papyrus, Imhotep describes examining a man with "a sprain in a vertebra of his spinal column." When he instructs the man to "Extend now thy two legs . . . he contracts them both immediately because of the pain he causes in the vertebra of his spinal column in which he suffers." The papyrus ends just as Imhotep begins to describe therapy for a low back sprain.

By Elizabethan times, such a sprain was considered a price of bawdiness, quite a trip from the biblical roots. Take, the example, the following lines from Shakespeare's *Measure for Measure*, when the prostitute, Mistress Overdone, enters:

Lucio. Behold, behold, where Madam Mitigation comes! I have
   purchased as many diseases under her roof as come to—
Second Gent. To what, I pray?
Lucio. Judge.
Second Gent. To three thousands dolours a year.
First Gent. Ay, and more.
Lucio. A French crown more.
First Gent. Thou art always figuring diseases in me; but thou art
   full of error: I am sound.
Lucio. Nay, not, as one would say, healthy; but so sound as things that
   are hollow: thy bones are hollow; impiety has made a feast of thee.
First Gent. How now! Which of your hips has the most profound
   sciatica?

Such metaphysical notions made little distinction between low back pain and sciatica. In the nineteenth century, anatomists and physicians started to make this distinction and to focus on disorders of the sciatic nerve itself as responsible for the pain radiating into the leg. The credit for entering the modern era goes to Charles Lasègue, who realized that the degree to which the leg was painful depended on the degree to which the nerve was stretched by various postures.[2] It fell to his students to describe the classic test for sciatica. Lasègue's Sign is the finding that flexing the extended leg at the hip provokes or exacerbates the pain. When the straight leg is bent at the hip beyond thirty degrees, the sciatic nerve is taut, which, for someone suffering from sciatica, provokes pain.

Railway Spine

Diseases that could be ascribed to the Industrial Revolution, from maiming to toxic exposures, blighted Victorian England. Even the railway, literally the engine of progress, caused concerns relating to derailment and the dangers of working on the railroad. But no ailment captured the public attention more than the recognition of "Railway Spine" in the 1860s. Railway Spine was not the fate of workers or customers involved in traumatic, violent accidents; it was the illness that could afflict passengers exposed to the vibrations and jostling of sitting in a moving passenger car.

The notion of such an illness found its champion in John Eric Erichsen, a young surgeon who by his early thirties had risen to the positions of professor at University College in London and surgeon to the Queen and had authored a comprehensive textbook, *The Science and Art of Surgery: A Treatise on Surgical Injuries, Diseases, and Operations* (1885). To Erichsen, it seemed reasonable that the spinal cord could suffer a "concussion" like the brain through even less physical trauma. In 1866 he published his collection of six essays on this topic in *Railway and Other Injuries of the Nervous System*. My personal copy is annotated by the original owner, one Thomas Pendle of Plymouth, who clearly found Erichsen's arguments compelling, as did many in British medicine and the public at large. Railway spine was a serious disorder. Pendle was particularly taken by Erichsen's ominous statement, "I have never known a patient to recover *completely and entirely, so as to be in the same state of health as before the accident*" (italics in original, p. 138). Riding the rails entailed the "rapidity of the movement, the momentum of the person injured, the suddenness of its arrest, the helplessness of the sufferers, and the natural perturbation of mind that must disturb the bravest . . . all circumstances that of a necessity greatly increase the severity of the resulting injury to the nervous system" (p. 9). All that jostling and jarring can result in "paralytic symptoms" that can last years. And indeed, growing numbers of passengers succumbed and even turned to the plaintiff's bar for remedy.

Erichsen inferred that the cause of this pervasive, chronic illness was a softening of the spinal cord, a molecular rearrangement. His inference was bolstered by his examination of these victims: "The state of the spine will be found to be the real cause of all these symptoms. On examining it by pressure, by percussion, or by the application of the hot sponge, it will be found that it is painful, and that its sensibility is exalted at one, two or three points . . . the upper cervical, the middle dorsal and the lumbar regions. . . . It is in consequence of the pain that . . . the spine loses its natural suppleness" (p. 102).

Erichsen initially held sway in Britain, but his notion engendered multiple counterarguments elsewhere, and soon critics emerged in Britain as well. The controversies over "Erichsen's Disease" played out over the next fifty years.[3] In Boston, G. L. Walton, professor of neurology at Harvard, was convinced early on that "railway spine" was a functional, behavioral disorder manifested as headache, insomnia, and irritability and was better labeled "Railway Brain." In Paris, Jean Martin Charcot, the famous neurologist and chief of the medical service at Salpêtrière, classified "railway spine" as a hysteria and ascribed the symptoms to "autosuggestion." Even Erichsen, shortly before his death in 1896, conceded that "neurosis" or "neurasthenia" were more appropriate pathophysiological theories than "concussion of the spine." It has been argued that this brouhaha was a boon to psychotherapy in that, in their rush to limit liability, surgeons and physicians employed by the railroads became psychotherapy's staunch advocates.[4] After all, the most influential textbook of medicine at the beginning of the twentieth century devoted a section to the "Traumatic Neuroses" and used "Railway Brain and Railway Spine" as object lessons as late as 1926.[5]

However, Railway Spine left a more lasting mark on the common sense. The notion that back pain can be part of a more pervasive, widespread, debilitating, and disabling illness is alive and well. So, too, is the notion that such an illness can be a consequence of minor trauma.

Ruptured Disc

The Industrial Revolution evolved at great human cost. For example, what was to become of a worker who was so severely injured he could not work? Was charity or life on the street the best society could offer? The late nineteenth-century workforce roiled with discontent and anger. Ferdinand Lassalle, Karl Marx, Upton Sinclair, Jack London, George Orwell, and many others gave voice to the anger. The union movement and the plaintiff's bar came to the fore. Revolution was in the air. From this ether, Otto von Bismarck emerged as the political genius who would squelch this unrest. Under his leadership, Prussia's legislature crafted a "welfare monarchy."[6]

The plan provided for universal health insurance. It was stratified when it came to disability awards, however. The worker who was injured on the job and incapable of work was deemed most worthy and qualified for wage replacement. The statute clearly targeted the worker who had suffered a violent workplace accident resulting in the loss of life or limb or some other grave injury. Work-related diseases, such as toxic exposures, were not covered by this legislation; other statutes would follow to that end.

From the outset, there were workers who claimed awards for less-catastrophic outcomes. "Telegraphist's Wrist" and "Writer's Cramp" became rallying cries of the labor unions and gained coverage in Britain and elsewhere early in the twentieth century, but not for long. These soon found themselves in the "traumatic neurosis" category with Railway Spine. And by this time, Railway Spine was more likely to be idling in tort litigation than bedeviling workers' compensation administrators.

All that changed in 1934. That's when a senior neurosurgeon and a junior orthopedist on the staff of the Massachusetts General Hospital invented the "ruptured disc."[7] Their scientific observation was that the center of the disc can extrude and impinge on local structures, but their more telling contribution was in the labeling. A rupture is a tearing apart; therefore, a rupture is an injury regardless of the cause. Every administrative-law judge working in workers' compensation jurisdictions pricked his ears. If a worker's regional backache was ascribed to a ruptured disc, the worker was "injured" on the job and covered under workers' compensation insurance.

Joseph Barr, the junior author on this seminal paper, wrote a paper twenty years later with the renowned Harvard psychiatrist John C. Nemiah acknowledging that he had been aware of the sociopolitical ramifications of the ruptured-disc label when it was invented and had come to regret the psychological consequences.[8] The experience of regional backache would never be the same.

So those of us with regional backache and those who treat it entered the twenty-first century with these three legacies:

1. The identification of a specific cause of backache, sciatica in particular, is highly pertinent.
2. Backache can be a sentinel symptom of a very widespread illness, which can be chronic and can result from minor trauma.
3. The physical demands of tasks that are customary and customarily comfortable can injure our back. After all, we can wear out our musculoskeletal system just as metals can fatigue.

These legacies are so entrenched as to be common sense. They color the experience of backache. They constrain clinical thinking. And they command public-health policy with a tenacity that spills over into many other issues. *Stabbed in the Back* attempts to advance the common sense so that it is commensurate with the state of the science and thereby facilitates a rational shift in the way we think about and react to low back pain and, ultimately, the way we construct and manage our health policy toward such ailments.

TWO

Oh, My Aching Back

The science of epidemiology has its roots in the study of epidemics and their causes. In classic epidemiology, something is observed—scurvy, for example—a causal hypothesis is generated, and the hypothesis is tested. Scottish physician James Lind made the connection between citrus fruit and the avoidance of scurvy. London doctor John Snow traced an outbreak of cholera in Soho to the common water tap. Making observations is easy. The proclivity for generating causal inferences is part of the human intellect. Recognizing which causal inferences can be tested is genius. Successfully testing them is science. Lind and Snow were scientists because they tested their hypotheses, Lind by prescribing limes and Snow by convincing the board of guardians of the parish to remove the handle from the Broad Street pump. Epidemics today, while rare though far from gone, remain the purview of epidemiology. A primary role for modern epidemiology evolved from this tradition of testing the putative causal exposure. Relying on cure as evidence for a causal association—or, short of cure, important improvement—has led to the development of the randomized controlled trial (RCT), which will occupy our attention in subsequent chapters.

Modern epidemiology has taken on a much broader agenda. Some of this agenda is descriptive epidemiology, which attempts to document the incidence (new cases in a given period of time) and prevalence (number of cases in the population at a point in time) of illnesses and diseases. To do so requires attention to the definition of the disease and the methodology for sampling any particular population. A third role for modern epidemiology is to determine whether perceived clinical associations are unlikely to happen by chance alone. To undertake these exercises, one must first define the outcome, the health effect, and the potential causes or exposures. Then one must design a study that tests whether any quantified relationship is as likely to occur by chance alone. If not, one is still left with uncertainty as to whether there is an influence or association that was not measured that can better explain the association. All epidemiology, but this form of exercise in particular, is at the mercy of two methodological marauders: bias and confounding.

Bias is the introduction of a systematic error into the measurement. An example of bias is "Berkson's Paradox." Berkson was a pioneering epidemiologist at the Mayo Clinic, which has two patient populations: the residents of surrounding Olmstead County and the patients referred from far and wide. Berkson realized that any two diseases were far more likely to occur in the same patient in the referral population than in the homegrown population. That's because the referrals are enriched for unusual presentations of disease, such as two diseases afflicting the same patient simultaneously.

Confounding is the influence of important factors that go unrecognized or unmeasured. For example, most fatal automobile accidents occur when driving between twenty-five and forty-five miles per hour. Before one assumes that driving either more slowly or more rapidly is safer, one needs to ask whether most driving occurs at twenty-five to forty-five miles per hour. It does. If one corrects for the likelihood of driving at any speed, the results are dramatically different: driving faster is far more dangerous.

Confounding and bias haunt all epidemiological studies. Furthermore, many associations are not univariate: it is seldom as simple as vitamin C and scurvy. For many conditions, the causal association is multivariate; age, socioeconomic status, education, body mass index, serum cholesterol, and much else that is known, unknown, and unknowable are causally associated with death from heart attacks. Measuring these, weighing their influence, and hoping that the most crucial confounders are not missed are the burdens of modern epidemiology. The study of low back pain has not been spared false conclusions because of inadequacies in study design, to say the least.

The Community Epidemiology of Backache

For generations, epidemiologists who studied backache and its treatment were wedded to convenience sampling. Convenience samples, also called ecological samples, are populations that are readily accessible; basically, they come to your office. Some of the epidemiologists were clinicians who considered their experience with their patients to be widely relevant. Some were interested in the insights they could derive from administrative data—the data accumulated by clinics, hospitals, governmental agencies, and insurers. Again, the belief was that these data defined what we know about back pain. The result was that what we thought we knew about back pain reflected the perspective of the observer, not the sufferer.

There are literally hundreds of thousands of papers putting forth inferences based on observations of the patients of a particular clinician, group of clinicians, clinic, or hospital. Erichsen's Railway Spine, discussed in the previous chapter, is a classic example. If Erichsen had bothered to go into East London, he would have found that probably 15 percent of the denizens would qualify for his diagnosis despite the fact that they had never traveled out of East London. Observational studies based on clinical experience have always suffered from an element of hubris: it is assumed that anyone in their right mind with a backache would seek care, so that what is observed in the clinic is the representation of the underlying disease. Hubris leads to a lack of concern about bias and confounding.

Observations based on clinical experience are not the only fog in the literature. Many more come from the records of insurance companies, hospitals, governments, and the like. These are even more "convenient," since one often need not even leave one's desk to gather the data. Conclusions derived from such data sets should be viewed as even more tenuous than inferences that derive from the clinic. Confounders and biases lurk there, too, and issues of accuracy are even greater. After all, the data have been collected and fit into the template furnished by the agency collecting the data. The collection and the templates are designed, generally, to serve billing and surveillance rather than the nuances of exposure and definitions of disease outcomes. Insurers are interested in the backache that is deemed an injury without regard to all the confounders that influence that certification. Workers' compensation data sets, for example, have very little in common with administrative data on admissions to hospitals or visits to clinics for backache.

Modern epidemiology recognizes the limited utility of convenience sampling and administrative data sets and designs studies that capture the experience of illness rather than its interface with recourse. Such studies demand that the investigators seek samples that are far from convenient. In community epidemiology, researchers go into the community and speak to the people in order to assess and define their experiences and to follow

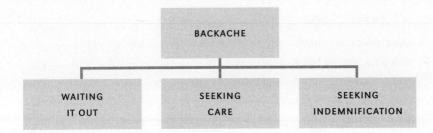

FIGURE 1. The predicament of regional low back pain

the course of their illnesses. The universe of people experiencing regional low back pain is illustrated in Figure 1. It includes those who suffer on their own, those who seek medical care, and those pursuing recourse for an "injury."

The Iceberg of Morbidity

Lois Verbrugge introduced the notion of the "iceberg of morbidity" over twenty years ago in arguing that convenience sampling revealed only a fraction of the ailments affecting the population at large. She was one of the investigators involved in the analysis of the Health in Detroit Survey, published in 1987.[1] The survey recruited a random sample of 600 adults willing to keep a diary. At the end of each day, they recorded any and all symptoms they experienced and what they did about them. Over a six-week period, women had some symptoms for nearly three weeks and men for about two, regardless of age. The most frequently cited symptoms were respiratory problems, followed closely by musculoskeletal problems. Half of these people experienced one or more musculoskeletal symptoms during the course of six weeks, and the typical symptom was likely to last a week. Pain was the most common musculoskeletal symptom by far, with stiffness a distant second. Furthermore, half of those afflicted were concerned that they were facing a serious problem. That's a lot of folks hurting out there in the community.

Back and upper-leg problems were the most common musculoskeletal symptoms, accounting for nearly half of all the problems recorded. All these episodes of regional musculoskeletal pain were transient. One would need to follow far more people for much longer than six weeks to capture anything more dire. Knee, neck, foot, and hand symptoms were similar in incidence and perhaps one-quarter as frequent as problems with the back and upper leg.

The Health in Detroit Survey was a daily diary study, and so it caught experiences that might otherwise have been quickly forgotten. Keeping such a record is a window into the normal challenges to our sense of well-being; it is why I commenced the introduction with, "To live a year without a backache is abnormal." To be well is not to permanently avoid backache (or other regional musculoskeletal disorders, let alone headache, heartache, heartburn, and much more). Such experiences are unavoidable in the course of life. To be well may not even require a coping style that incorporates denying or ignoring the problem. To be well requires some personal resources that facilitate effective coping. This last insight is bolstered by other exercises in community epidemiology.

Variations in Recall of Backache

From diary studies such as the Health in Detroit Survey, we know that regional backache is a frequent, ubiquitous, and intermittent predicament of life. Any survey based on a less-immediate measure is tapping into the reliability of recall of recent and prior episodes. Dozens of community surveys in the United States and elsewhere have targeted the experience of low back pain. There is a degree of commonality to the inferences derived from these studies. However, even more striking is the variability of the results. Some reflect differences in the survey methodology. It matters greatly if one inquires about backache in the past week, or month, or quarter, or year. The longer the interval, the more our recall is telescoped into recent months or weeks. It also matters how backache is described in the survey. Does the query capture just discrete low back pain or pain that is more generalized, pain that is disabling, pain associated with absenteeism from work, pain that sent one to the doctor, and so forth? Each of these nuances will alter the population sampled, but they are not the most critical determinants of the results of these surveys. The most critical determinants relate to the psychosocial complexion of the population being surveyed. Rather than present a compendium of these studies, I will focus on a few that are exemplary and telling.

The National Health Interview Survey (NHIS) has long been conducted by the Centers for Disease Control and Prevention, the National Center for Health Statistics, and the U.S. Census Bureau. Each year a representative sample of households across the United States is selected. Each selected household is contacted by letter, and a trained interviewer visits to administer the survey in person. The survey asks a wide range of questions aiming to define the "health" of the nation. Tucked into the survey is a question relating to the occurrence of back pain in the past three months that lasted at least a day and was not trivial. In the 2002 survey, which sampled 31,000 adults older than eighteen, approximately 17 percent reported isolated low back pain in the previous three months.[2] Extrapolated to the population as a whole, over 15 million adult Americans suffer low back pain every three months. Table 1 presents the descriptive statistics. As one can see, 14 to 20 percent of Americans in many categories could recall a day or more of low back pain in the past three months. That means that most of the people recording a week of backache in their diaries in the Health in Detroit Survey would have no recall six weeks later. But many, perhaps a third, would.

There is a limit to how much more one can meaningfully infer from the descriptive statistics in Table 1. For example, older Americans and retired Americans are more likely to report back pain than younger adults who never worked. This may have nothing to do with exposures at work, though, as retired workers are likely to be older and older people retired, so aging may be the more determinative factor. Likewise, certain related variables might account for the increased prevalence in whites compared to minorities. There are statistical methods, forms of multivariate analysis, that can correct for the influence of one variable on another. Furthermore, multivariate analyses allow one to look for associations of the report of back pain with particular medical conditions or with psychological conditions and health-averse behaviors—associations that cannot be accounted for by the sociodemographic characteristics in Table 1 or by other variables that are assessed in the survey.

It turns out that the people reporting low back pain are more likely to have other important medical conditions, often an assortment of such. They also are more likely to be overweight and to abuse tobacco and alcohol. The descriptor "more likely" is too open-ended to stand without definition. These multivariate analyses lend themselves to the calculation of a ratio of the prevalence of low back pain to the variable under consideration. This is usually expressed as an "odds ratio," which may not be the exact number but is in the range that is unlikely to occur by chance alone (the "95 percent confidence interval"). For coincident medical conditions (comorbidities) and health-averse behaviors, the odds ratio is around 1.3, with confidence intervals ranging from 1.1 to 1.5. That means that anyone reporting back pain is a bit more likely, perhaps 30 percent more likely, to also report another major medical condition or health-averse behavior. So

TABLE 1. Associations with Prevalent Low Back Pain
in the 2002 National Health Interview Survey

CHARACTERISTIC	SUBGROUP	PERCENTAGE
Total Population		17.0
Age Group	18–24	5.0
	24–34	15.9
	35–44	16.2
	45–54	17.3*
	55–64	18.6*
	>65	19.7*
Sex	Male	16.5
	Female	17.6*
Race/ethnicity	White, non-Hispanic	17.9
	Black, non-Hispanic	15.6*
	Other, non-Hispanic	14.2*
	Hispanic	14.1*
Education	Less than high school	18.5
	High school or GED	17.8
	Some college	17.5
	Bachelor/associate degree	15.9*
	More than bachelor degree	14.0*
Marital status	Married	17.3
	Previously married	18.7*
	Never married	14.3*
	Unmarried couple	19.3
Employment status	Currently working	15.9
	Retired	19.9*
	Formerly worked	20.0*
	Never worked	12.9*

Source: T. W. Strine and J. M. Hootman, "U.S. National Prevalence and Correlates of Low Back
and Neck Pain among Adults," Arthritis and Rheumatism (Arthritis Care and Research) 57
(2007): 656–65.

*Statistically significantly different from the first level of each subgroup

56.5 percent of people who denied back or neck pain in the previous three months were considered overweight, whereas 64.3 percent of those with back pain were overweight. This is a small absolute difference—8 percent—that would occur by chance infrequently. If the difference was larger and therefore the odds ratio greater, it is less likely that a confounder is lurking, some covariate that one did not or could not measure. Perhaps the more overweight individuals, who are more likely to have many diseases, are more accustomed to and more comfortable with reporting all sorts of life predicaments. Rather than having more backache, the overweight are more attuned to remembering it. That may just be a guess, but it is not that fatuous of a confounder. For that reason, most of us are cautious about hanging our hats on odds ratios less than 2.0, particularly when the absolute difference is small.

Another set of associations teased out of the NHIS dealt with psychological factors (Table 2). A picture is emerging from surveys such as the NHIS of the quality of life of the subset of the population that recalls important low back pain. Members of that group tend to have more health problems, manifest more health-averse behaviors, and be more likely to be living under a pall. However, the NHIS is a cross-sectional study, a snapshot of the population at one point in time. It offers no insight into temporality; it does not clarify which factor is the cart and which is the horse. Are these people sad because their backs hurt, or are they more likely to recall the last episode of backache because they are sad and have difficulty ignoring any further challenge to their sense of well-being? Cross-sectional studies cannot answer this question. One would need to have a different study design, a longitudinal study, which follows people over time and which is far more demanding of investigators.

Hence, cross-sectional studies are more frequently undertaken. They offer a quick and convenient method for probing for possible associations. Many countries have undertaken surveys similar to the NHIS over the years. Because of the role back pain plays in work absenteeism, the British have long conducted postal surveys probing the prevalence of back pain lasting twenty-four hours or longer during the previous year and its relationship to occupational factors. When the survey conducted in 1987–88 was compared to the survey conducted a decade later, it was noted that the prevalence of back pain increased from 36 percent to 49 percent, although backache of such severity that the person couldn't put on hosiery did not increase.[3] This rising prevalence in the recall of backache in the

TABLE 2. Psychological Factors Associated with Prevalent Back Pain
in the 2002 National Health Interview Survey

CHARACTERISTIC	ODDS RATIO (95% CONFIDENCE INTERVAL)
All or most of the time in past 30 days	
So sad, nothing could cheer you up	1.5 (1.2–2.0)
Nervous	1.9 (1.5–2.2)
Restless and fidgety	1.7 (1.5–2.0)
Hopeless	1.5 (1.1–1.9)
Everything is an effort	1.8 (1.5–2.2)
Likely cases of serious mental illness	1.8 (1.5–2.3)

Source: T. W. Strine and J. M. Hootman, "U.S. National Prevalence and Correlates of Low Back and Neck Pain among Adults," Arthritis and Rheumatism (Arthritis Care and Research) 57 (2007): 656–65.

Note: All of these odds ratios are statistically adjusted to account for all the sociodemographic variables in Table 1 as well as comorbidities. All are statistically significant since the confidence interval does not cross 1.0. If it did, then the odds ratio is sufficiently likely to be unity that the possibility of a difference in prevalence should be taken with a grain of salt. Nonetheless, these are marginal odds ratios in terms of magnitude.

community was no surprise, as the number of patient visits for backache and the number of days of sick leave ascribed to backache had been rising as dramatically, leading one British epidemiologist to query, "Is life becoming more of a pain?"[4] He went on to posit that the explanation for the increased prevalence of back pain was due to a number of factors, including the more sedentary lives of the sufferers, distress and dissatisfaction in daily life, and increasing public attention to the ailment.

As epidemic as back pain is becoming in Britain, the prevalence is much higher in Germany.[5] This observation was made utilizing data from a Europe-wide study of osteoporosis. Pain in the low back is not what is varying across countries. Rather, the experience of illness and the idioms chosen by the afflicted in offering a narrative of their illness experience is tempered by "sociocultural influences" that vary from country to country. The pain in the low back may not differ between the German citizenry and the British, but the illness that is engendered by that pain clearly does.

Medicine is one driving force in fashioning "sociocultural influences" that contribute to the experience of illness, but medicine, too, is subject to sociopolitical constraints, many of which are legislated. As I mentioned in chapter 1, at the turn of the twentieth century, the Prussian legislature created a welfare monarchy (*Reichsversicherungsordnung*). Such ideas as national health insurance, workers' compensation insurance, Social Security disability schemes, and impairment-based disability are a Prussian legacy. The post–World War II German economic boom (*Wirtschaftswunder*) took the principles of the welfare monarchy to extremes Lassalle or even Marx could not have imagined. Most economists focus on Germany's eight weeks of vacation as excessive. I have no problem if Germany can afford such indulgence. As a student of illness and its behaviors, however, I have been troubled by the German entitlement to rehabilitation. A decade ago, at the time of the osteoporosis survey,[6] Germans were eligible for as much as a month a year of various forms of spa therapy for ailments that are common in the course of normal living, albeit commonly daunting. Medicalizing such ailments, while seemingly empathic, challenges one's concept of wellness. A backache that might have been considered a nuisance is likely to be considered an illness worthy of recall and possibly treatment. Backache in Germany became something people must endure, pending therapy in a spa; elsewhere it remained more of an intermittent predicament with which one must cope. The results of the survey suggest that many German people inculcated a narrative of illness, of "Oh, my aching back," between palliative visits to the spa. In recent years, bowing to economic realities, the German government has reduced this entitlement, but Germany's backache history remains a textbook case of the way societal choices can influence the perception of illness among the population.

THREE

The Pall of Persistence

As I hope I have convinced you, regional low back pain is an intermittent and recurring predicament of life. Episodes vary in intensity and duration, and the periods in between episodes vary both in degree of remission and duration. For some, the wait for improvement may seem interminable. Cross-sectional studies can do little to explore the persistence of the pain; that requires a longitudinal study. There are several such cohort studies.

The Saskatchewan Health and Back Pain Survey was a one-year postal survey conducted in the late 1990s.[1] If you follow a cohort of adults who recalled no back pain in the six months prior to the beginning of the study and ask them at six months and one year if they recall back pain, about 19 percent will answer in the affirmative. That means the annual incidence of low back pain is 19 percent. Most episodes were mild and transient. For 1 percent, the pain was "intense," and half of those found it disabling. But this study design offers little insight into the recurrence of episodes.

For that we can turn to studies such as the Canadian National Population Health Survey (NPHS), which is similar to the NHIS discussed in the previous chapter but lends itself to longitudinal studies because it revisits the same people repeatedly. The NPHS included an incidence study similar to the Saskatchewan Health and Back Pain Survey, but the query was not the development of any back pain but the following: "Have you been diagnosed by a health professional with . . . long-term [back] problems?," defined as lasting or expected to last six months or longer. The incidence of this degree of back problems was about 5 percent.[2]

Once afflicted with persistent back pain of this nature, a person has little likelihood of experiencing remission. Rather, he or she is at risk of joining the subculture of those with chronic back pain. A number of years ago, my colleagues and I interviewed by telephone a random sample of nearly 4,500 civilian, noninstitutionalized North Carolina residents age twenty-one and older.[3] In the year prior to the interview, 3.9 percent had suffered back pain that limited usual activities continuously for three or more months or had been through twenty-five or more episodes of pain. Most of these individuals considered their general health far from good; a third reported that they were permanently disabled by back pain. Most sought medical care, many sought alternative care, and most had taken to bed more than once because of back pain. These people should be thought of as a special subset of low-back-pain sufferers rather than an extreme of the range of usual back pain. In community epidemiology, they are generally denoted as having "chronic back pain." In the clinical literature, they are the "chronic back" patients, "failed back" patients, and claimants for indemnity awards for disabling back pain or compensable back "injuries." Theirs is a sorry lot in the clinic. In this chapter, we are exploring their experience at home and in the community.

Persistent Widespread Pain

Epidemiology has only recently come to understand the plight of those in the community who are suffering persistent back pain. Part of the reason for the delay is that much of the early work focused on particular anatomical regions, such as chronic low back pain or neck pain or knee pain. The breakthrough came when epidemiologists started to enquire whether anyone with persistent pain in a particular part of the body also had pain elsewhere. Multisite pain turns out to be the rule, with the low back the most frequent site. A recent postal survey of a sample of patients enrolled in sixteen general practices in southeastern England is illustrative and representative of similar surveys in many countries.[4]

The survey was as comprehensive as several we have already visited. Persistent musculoskeletal pain was defined as pain for more than half the days in the last year in any of thirteen musculoskeletal sites. A person was defined as having persistent multisite pain if he or she affirmed such pain in two or more sites. The study defined a person as having "chronic widespread pain" if he or she had pain for at least three months in at least two sections of two limbs on opposite sides of the body and in the "axial skeleton" (medicalspeak for the spine). Nearly half the people surveyed had persistent musculoskeletal pain, of which 25 percent had pain in a single site, 52 percent in two to four sites, 18 percent in five to seven sites,

TABLE 3. Multivariate Analysis of the Relationship between Persistent Musculoskeletal Pain and Sociodemographic Characteristics in the Southeast England Postal Survey

ASSOCIATIONS	ODDS RATIO (95% CONFIDENCE INTERVAL)
Single-site chronic pain	
Male gender	1.4 (1.1–1.9)
Psychological distress	0.7 (0.5–1.0)
High disability	0.7 (0.4–1.2)
High pain intensity	0.6 (0.4–0.8)
Chronic widespread pain	
Male gender	0.5 (0.4–0.7)
Under 56 years	0.5 (0.4–0.7)
Psychological distress	1.9 (1.4–2.6)
High disability	1.4 (1.0–2.1)
High pain intensity	4.0 (2.9–5.5)
Multisite chronic pain	
Male gender	0.8 (0.7–1.0)
Under 56 years	0.5 (0.4–0.6)
Psychological distress	1.8 (1.4–2.2)
High disability	1.4 (0.9–2.0)
High pain intensity	5.2 (4.1–6.7)

Source: D. Carnes, S. Parsons, D. Ashby, A. Breen, N. E. Foster, T. Pincus, S. Vogel, and M. Under-wood, "Chronic Musculoskeletal Pain Rarely Presents in a Single Body Site: Results for the UK Population Study," Rheumatology 46 (2007): 1168–70.

Note: An odds ratio is indicative of an increased likelihood of the association when the confidence interval does not bracket 1.0. The likelihood is considered robust if the odds ratio itself exceeds 2.0.

and 4 percent in more than eight sites. A multivariate analysis was performed, probing for associations between categories of persistent pain and some of the other variables assessed in the survey. The principal results are presented in Table 3.

Persistent single-site pain, often low back pain, is more likely to afflict men and to be considered moderately intense. Multisite pain and chronic widespread pain are more likely to afflict younger women who manifest more general psychological distress and perceive the pain as highly intense. The person with chronic widespread pain is a tragic figure, one that has commanded a good deal of attention in the past decade. These sad and hurting people constitute 5 to 10 percent of the population in most surveys. Chronic widespread pain is the fate of most caught in the vortex of disability determination for their persistent back pain. I argue that "chronic widespread pain" is the appropriate categorization for clinical as well as community epidemiology. My argument has yet to carry the day, however. Rather, the current label is "fibromyalgia." The notion of fibromyalgia has found a wide lay audience. It also supports the practices of some providers of medical and alternative therapies while remaining a point of confusion if not contention in medicine in general. It merits detailed discussion here. Many of the concepts relevant to the notion of fibromyalgia are also relevant to the experience of persistent and chronic low back pain in the chapters that follow.

The Social Construction of Fibromyalgia

Molière penned the aphorism "Doubts are more cruel than the worst of truths" in *Le Misanthrope* over three centuries ago. This idea is so central to the Western philosophy of life that it intrudes into our most intimate moments. It is always present in the doctor-patient relationship. We now know that the ideation of uncertainty can lead to alterations in physiology that compromise health and longevity. Uncertainty can be morbid and mortal . . . and pathogenic. "Fibromyalgia" is the object lesson.

"Fibromyalgia" is an assertion of uncertainty. The pathogenesis of this illness is closely associated with the quest for its cause. People with persistent widespread pain need to understand this when they "choose" to be patients, and physicians need to learn to diminish the harmfulness. Persistent widespread pain is not a disease of pathobiology. Despite a concerted effort for some time, no abnormality in any organ system has been identified as associated with fibromyalgia, nor does one become manifest during its prolonged course. Absence of proof of a pathobiological cause, of course, is not proof of its absence. Some clinical investigators continue to pursue this will-o'-the-wisp with enthusiasm that far outstrips the yield. Perhaps there is no biologic abnormality. Fibromyalgia is a learned illness, taught over time by a number of actors, including physicians. Fibromyalgia patients are in desperate search for a label that is acceptable to society at large and its agents of credibility: the media, the insurance industry, and the pharmaceutical industry. Fibromyalgia is a symbol of the diagnostic process gone awry.

The Semiotics of Illness

The tradition of scholarship that takes the role of medicine in society as its subject is rooted in semiotics, the branch of philosophy that considers the meaning of signs and symbols. Scholars have approached the semiotics of illness from the perspectives of philosophy, history, anthropology, sociology, jurisprudence, and other disciplines. Some familiarity with several of the precepts is prerequisite to understanding the process that is fibromyalgia.

Social Constructions

Ideas that have gained general credence are the fabric of daily living. They are nurtured by a network of believers. They are peculiar to particular societies at particular times in their history. Race, normal sexual behavior, kinship, and authorship are notions that have proved mutable in recent memory. Since each of these ideas is created by particular individuals, reflecting particular intellectual, economic, and other interests and operating in particular historical contexts, they are often termed "social constructions." Defining the boundary between fact, or "truth," and social construction has driven epistemology for centuries and is hotly debated today.[5] For me, the boundary is artificial; everything is real and everything is socially constructed. Without social constructions, chaos would reign. Social constructions define the rules of community. Most are not "bad."

Seldom does a social construction stand without challenge, at least not for long. The challenge is most often in the form of an alternative construction. When a particular iteration is generally believed to be correct, alternatives are relegated to the fringe. For a more deviant construction to survive disdain and other social pressures, the zeal of its makers in recruiting a network of adherents must be inexhaustible.

For the health-care professions, "common practice" is the parallel to social constructions. Common practice is as mutable as any social construction; witness the evolution of the definitions of "aggressive" versus "conservative" therapies in one generation of physicians. Conservative approaches, once considered rational, came to be regarded as nihilistic, while aggressive approaches, formerly considered marginal or unconscionable, were lauded. For common practice to persist, the advocacy of committed practitioners is required. So it is that one profession (spine surgeons) can extol "laminectomy" (removal of the lamina portion of the vertebral bone) for backache with the same certainty that another (chiropractic) can extol "adjusting subluxations." Not only do the proponents hold firmly to their beliefs, but their patients also can be zealous in that regard.

The creed of contemporary medicine is that science trumps consensus and advocacy in honing common practice. Clearly, some common practices have yielded to systematic testing that proves them flawed. Equally clearly, some common practices do not lend themselves to scientific refutation, and for others the voices of the advocates overwhelm their lack of scientific support. Such advocacy takes strength from inferential arguments (the practice is plausible, outcomes seem consistent, and the like) and gains momentum from the degree to which it advantages the advocates and seduces their clientele. This dialectic supports many a "complementary" or "alternative" health-care system. It also supports many a medical practice, notably the diagnosis and treatment of fibromyalgia. The seductiveness of any unproved, perhaps unprovable common medical practice reflects the degree to which hubris has been inculcated by the training of the physician. Hence, the committed practitioner can reframe fibromyalgia as a biological disease. Labeling becomes the salve for uncertainty, if not anguish, for any who are suffering from persistent widespread pain.

Medicalization and Illness Behaviors

Medicalization is the act of framing life experiences as medical or clinical or pathobiological. For some life experiences, the framing is perfectly rational (crushing chest pain, for example). However, for many life experiences, such framing reflects preconceptions, myths, tenuous inferences, marketing, and other influences on the common sense. In the past forty years, it has become clear that medicalization of some life experiences carries with it a considerable downside, often enough so that the notion of medicalization has come to carry extensive baggage and the term has become pejorative. Some personal attributes have been considered unusual, aberrant, or deviant, depending on whether they were framed in the context of moral transgression or in the context of disease. If the attribute is considered a moral problem, it is secularized. If the attribute is defined as a disease, it is medicalized. Suicide and particular sexual proclivities have spent generations in one or the other of these arenas. In recent decades, homosexuality has been secularized and alcoholism has been medicalized by both medical and legal decree; obesity has been medicalized by medical decree, with some wobbling in the conviction.

Up until the late seventeenth century, medical diagnoses were simply a categorization of symptoms. Then Thomas Sydenham outlined a system of classifying diseases by focusing on their symptoms.[6] This revolutionary system made it possible for physicians to infer the disorder of anatomy or physiology (the disease) that was causing any set of symptoms (the illness). (For example, fever is not a freestanding disease but a symptom of illness stemming from several possible illnesses.) This disease-illness paradigm was a monumental conceptual watershed for medicine. Without Sydenham's insight, there would be textbooks on "agues" instead of on infectious diseases.

In the early twentieth century, medicine applied Sydenham's paradigm to a new realm, one as the arbiter of which *behaviors* were consonant with particular *disease* states. Physicians assumed responsibility for medicalizing work absenteeism and long-term disability. Medicalization as a social force reached its peak in the 1970s. Symptoms that were considered to be consonant with a particular disease were deemed "real," as opposed to deviant or "functional complaints," or "illness behaviors." The chroniclers and analysts of this dialectic include Eliot Freidson,[7] who spoke of medicine's "professional dominance," and Paul Starr,[8] who proclaimed its "cultural authority." This is a cultural hegemony that turned physicians into moral entrepreneurs. Among the moral entrepreneurs were crusaders for clinical matters viewed as crucial to the health of the public, or to a segment of the public, even if the view was a construction of illness based solely on conviction.[9]

The organization of U.S. medicine has changed dramatically in the past thirty years, but its cultural hegemony has not. Medicalization today encompasses a range of human conditions, from ill-behaving children to people whose sleep habits are defined as abnormal and the misery of chronic widespread pain. Regarding the latter, on June 30, 1999, a resolution was introduced in the U.S. House of Representatives (HR 237 IH) recognizing "the severity of the issue of fibromyalgia" and defining it as a "chronic disorder characterized by widespread musculoskeletal pain and tenderness" that "may be triggered by stress, trauma, or possibly an infectious agent in susceptible people."

The Sick Role

Sydenham's legacy is a system of medicine that considers disease its *raison d'être*. The successes are legion. If it were not for his illness-disease dualism, modern medicine would be treating catarrh rather than fashioning specific cures for pneumonias. However, the successes are so impressive that the illness-disease paradigm has become the first and primary recourse for nearly every personal predicament; a scientific solution will be forthcoming if the patient and physician collaborate in the exercise of defining the underlying disease. What happens if the disease or the cure is elusive? This caveat is seldom raised in a culture that values curing the disease, but it is particularly relevant to all who see no better option than to be patients for predicaments they perceive to be abnormal but that others consider normal.

Clinical investigators, medical anthropologists, and others have long probed this caveat. This science lacks cachet because it focuses not on disease but on the experience of illness. It is often criticized as "nonscientific" or "observational" or "inductive," to which I counter: so is much that passes for "scientific." At least the scholars of the illness experience acknowledge the limitations of studying illness. After all, people vary in many ways, including dramatically in the fashion in which they experience illness. No rules of illness behaviors will ever apply universally. Many of the pioneers of the study of the illness experience held sway half a century ago, when "hard science" was barely an establishment. One was David Mechanic, who wrote: "Illness behavior—the manner in which people differentially perceive, evaluate and respond to symptoms—may be viewed from at least three general perspectives. Such patterns of behavior may be seen (a) as a product of social and cultural conditioning, (b) as part of a coping repertoire, or (c) in terms of their usefulness for the patient who obtains certain advantages from the 'sick role.'"[10] Mechanic was a student of the importance of whether and why people recognize symptoms, make contacts with doctors, accept or reject advice about treatment, and remain under or discontinue medical supervision, particularly in response to various types of pain and placebo reactions. He recognized the ways in which cultural and social pressures influence an individual's recognition that she or he needs advice. Mechanic did not consider "illness behaviors" aberrant. Illness is never suffered in the abstract. Illness is an intimate companion to be confronted, and in the confronting one must adapt behavior that would not be necessary if one were well, even the behavior of acting as if one were well. All illness induces behavioral adaptation. The adaptation is a function of preconceived notions and sociological precedents playing upon one's personal psychological makeup.

Illness behaviors may be productive in that they enhance coping, diminish the impact of the illness, lead others to empathize with the sufferer, and drive beneficial choices. Illness behaviors can be counterproductive when they impede coping or healing or elicit adverse behavior in providers and caregivers. This counterproductive behavior is what is generally labeled as "illness behavior," but that, too, is a construction. We should speak of "adaptive" and "maladaptive" illness behaviors and abandon the chauvinism that assumes the adapting takes the physician and not the illness as the point of reference. What may seem maladaptive to the treating physician in the context of the treatment act might simply reflect the rules of engagement, which are often superimposed by various stakeholders.

The maladaptive illness behaviors that are characteristic of patients with chronic disabling regional musculoskeletal disorders are, in all likelihood, a predictable result of the regulated process of disability determination.[11] The process is designed to question the veracity of the patient's claim of disabling pain in a setting where a validating underlying disease is elusive. The development of maladaptive illness behaviors reflects a desperate, often angry response by the patient to not being believed.[12] It is maladaptive from the perspective of the physicians who are sitting in judgment. It is often maladaptive for the treating physicians and even the claimant's caring community. But for the claimant, it is adaptive, in that it preserves some sense of self, including some sense of self-efficacy. The maladaptive illness behaviors are not symptoms of pain; they are symptoms of suffering.[13] That is as true of patients labeled as having fibromyalgia as it is of claimants/patients labeled as having chronic back pain, a failed back, or disabling back pain.

Illness behaviors have many dimensions. They have a verbal dimension in terms of the narrative of distress that the patient chooses to, or learns to, articulate. That narrative is always laced with idioms that are learned and used to mark the experience. Much is learned in the course of treatment. Physicians can silence their patients and rescript their narratives, thereby causing their medical self-stories to conform to a preconceived notion of the manifestations of any given disease. Patients with rheumatoid arthritis become comfortable responding to queries as to the duration of morning stiffness but are less comfortable responding to a request for a "pain score" without modifying the request as to when and which joint. Patients with chronic regional musculoskeletal disorders learn to score their pain as global and acquire idioms of distress that are peculiar to this clinical situation. Patients labeled with fibromyalgia, when compared to patients with rheumatoid arthritis, express pessimistic beliefs about themselves and others, assuming the worst possible outcomes.[14] They consider themselves more ill than do those suffering from emphysema, rheumatoid arthritis, or even advanced cancer.[15] For these patients, fibromyalgia is no social construction; it has transformed into real, pervasive, awful bodily sensations.

The Semiotics of Fibromyalgia

Every diagnostic label is an exercise in semiotics:

> No one *has* fibromyalgia.
> No one suffers *from* fibromyalgia.
> There are patients who suffer fibromyalgia.

Fibrositis would probably have remained on the medical fringe were it not for the initiative in the mid-1980s by Merck, Sharp and Dohme, Inc., to expand the indications for cyclobenzaprine hydrochloride (Flexeril), its novel putative muscle relaxant, to the disorder. Merck partially underwrote the machinations of a "committee" of the American College of Rheumatology, which supplanted "fibrositis" with the "fibromyalgia" label and drafted the vaunted "1990 Criteria for the Classification of Fibromyalgia."[16] In addition to persistent widespread pain, a patient had to have an exquisite aversion to being poked in at least eleven of eighteen specified anatomical sites to qualify for the fibromyalgia label. The criteria have weathered poorly. That is not surprising, since they are the product of circular reasoning: they were derived from the same population from which the hypothesis was generated. The quantification of tender points has proved such a sophistry that even the lead author of the criteria has decried their use in the clinic.[17] Absent "tender points," the criteria suggest that anyone with persistent widespread pain qualifies for labeling as suffering from fibromyalgia.

The promulgation of criteria under the imprimatur of the American College of Rheumatology was a crucial moment in the history of the construction of fibromyalgia. It legitimated fibromyalgia in the eyes of many clinicians and the medicolegal establishment. It has vindicated patients whose misery was confounded by the many who doubted that symptoms could be "real" in the absence of demonstrable disease. It has led to an explosion in the diagnosis. And it has caused a number of investigators to turn their attention to the epidemiology of persistent widespread pain.

People suffering persistent widespread pain are more likely to be mired in the lower socioeconomic strata,[18] to be unhappy and anxious,[19] and to suffer symptoms they interpret as indicating that more than their musculo-skeletal system is diseased.[20] They feel compelled to frequent primary-care practices the world round, although whether they are considered depressed or just unhappy depends on the prevailing social constructions regarding affective states.[21] Most will not qualify for labeling as a sufferer of a primary affective disorder,[22] although the affect of many is distinctive.[23]

Fortunately, some relief is in sight for most sufferers of persistent wide-spread pain. Their natural history, with or without the ministrations of caregivers, is one of waxing and waning,[24] although they are not likely to become pain free.[25] This is particularly unlikely if they attend rheumatol-ogy clinics that specialize in fibromyalgia.[26] Of course, this last observation cannot reliably be construed to impugn the ministrations of the rheuma-tologists in these clinics. After all, it may be that referrals are biased toward patients who are more ill. Neither can it be reliably construed that the rheu-matology patients have a distinctive form of persistent widespread pain. All the descriptive community-based epidemiology summarized above is more consistent with a range of individual differences in the experience of regional musculoskeletal pain rather than distinctive subsets. A similar conclusion can be drawn from analyses of the attributes of people with persistent widespread pain who elect to, or feel they have no other option than to, become patients with fibromyalgia.[27] What distinguishes people in the community with persistent widespread pain from patients with fibro-myalgia is the magnitude of psychological distress associated with the pain rather than its degree of painfulness. People with persistent widespread pain choose to seek care when the "painfulness" is insufferable and no other recourse seems as reasonable.

If chronic persistent pain is within the range of normal human expe-riences, albeit at the unpleasant extreme, is it abnormal? If it is an ex-perience that the person finds tolerable, or tolerable for a time, is that person abnormal? There are telling analogies. For example, if one is per-sisting at great personal cost, at great personal "pain" if you will, in an unsatisfactory intimate relationship or job, should we label that person abnormal? Epidemiology is hard-pressed to define such boundaries; there are simply too many variables. If there is an operational definition, it is that the suffering is insufferable to the sufferer or for those in the sufferer's intimate community. Persistent widespread pain is rendered insufferable by an abnormal convergence of personal and societal influences. Efforts at palliation need to confront the influences that caused the pain to be insufferable as assiduously as they confront the pain itself, if not more so.

This approach to palliation runs counter to the usual patient-physician contract that takes the definition and treatment of the "disease" as its charge. What therapeutic contract can be initiated with a complaint of "I can't stand it any longer" and elicit the diagnosis, "Your pain is insufferable"? What do we call the state of medically inexplicable yet personally insufferable physical pain? This is not the kind of pain, or pain state, that is reflexively aversive, responsive to painkillers, and difficult to express in language or even unspeakable.[28] This is an emotive state that is unresponsive to painkillers[29] and provokes dramatic narratives of distress. As we will see, it is also the fate of so many with chronic back pain who are trapped in the vortex of disability determination. Drugs offer little benefit in the setting of a disorder such as fibromyalgia that is a social construction rather than a disease.[30]

Hypochondria

Fibromyalgia is a latecomer in the labeling of people whose symptoms elude ready explanation. Labeling has reflected all sorts of religious, metaphysical, psychological, and physiologic perspectives.[31] In the early nineteenth century, French histologist Marie Francois Bichat put forward the idea that human beings were divided into two "lives." The "vegetative" life was inherent to the viscera, painful, and seated in the abdomen under the ribs (the hypochondrium). The "animal" life was interactive and conscious. Hypochondriasis resulted when forces moved vegetative sensations into consciousness. Today, hypochondriasis denotes patients who are preoccupied with the pervasive fear and unshakable belief that they have a serious, undiagnosed disease accounting for their physical sensations. They are patients who *somatize*, who focus on the physical manifestations of emotional distress.[32]

"Somatization"[33] is the legacy of psychosomatics, a psychoanalytic theory that came to prominence in the middle of the twentieth century.

The initial postulate was that psychic conflict can provoke organ dysfunction. Today, somatization is the suggestion that symptoms of organ dysfunction rather than organ dysfunction itself can be the expression of emotions. Implicit in this concept is the belief that the expression of emotions as bodily symptoms is abnormal and acknowledgment of such is prerequisite to "cure." Abandoning all these notions is long overdue. Somatization is one of the "normal" patterns of self-awareness, one of the personality quirks that many live with quite successfully. Somatization is a problem only when it becomes sufficiently distressful.

Everyone who is suffering distressful somatic perceptions casts about for a reason, for a rationale to frame their experience as disease.[34] In times long past, moral turpitude and diabolical possessions were plausible. In the Industrial Revolution, just riding in a railway car was a plausible explanation for the pervasive illness labeled Railway Spine. Today, even Congress has gotten involved in attributing causes of persistent widespread pain. The contemporary social construction has thoroughly medicalized insufferable somatic perceptions. To suggest to these sufferers that their suffering is a functional somatic syndrome—a "somatoform disorder" with psychological roots—will predictably elicit resentment, often anger, and rarely prove helpful. The patient is prepared to be medicalized and not to hear that the symptoms are "in the mind" and therefore either evidence of a mental illness or a form of confabulation.[35]

The therapeutic issue today is not the label, not even the uncertainty arising from the fact that the symptoms cannot be medically explained.[36] The challenge is to breach the dominant construction of pain as disease. Then the therapeutic issue becomes the social and psychological factors that compromise coping to the degree that the symptoms are rendered insufferable. Ingvar Hazemeijer and Johannes Rasker term this the "therapeutic domain."[37] The therapeutic challenge is to tear down the social constructions to address this issue. Mechanic understood this over forty years ago.[38]

The Neurophysiology of Insufferable Persistent Widespread Pain

Just as the epidemiology of health progressed in the past decade, so too has the neurophysiology of pain. The advances of earlier decades largely dealt with the way the nervous system recognizes that something is painful at the source of the pain, such as the neurology that causes us to reflexively pull our hand off a hot pot. Awareness of the event and emotional responses to the event were seen to be secondary to the sensory input. In the past decade, neurophysiologists have been rethinking this model. A "constructivist" theory has emerged suggesting that awareness is a result of parallel neurologic processes that build our personal reality from the sensory input. This theory of constructivism recruits memory, prior experiences, and genetic differences in neurologic responsiveness to the conditioning of the painful stimulus as it emerges into our consciousness.

There is no doubt that neurophysiologic constructs of this nature also account for much that metaphysics considered the "mind" and the "soul." Our emotions, our educational accomplishments, our tightly held beliefs, and much more reflect neurophysiologic constructs. The fashion in which we respond to life's joys and life's challenges reflects the idiosyncratic nature of these constructs. There is also no doubt that this is true of acute and chronic stress and distress, with consequences that can be more dramatic than simply changes in our neuroendocrine physiology. There is a wide range of individual difference, of inherited difference, in this biology, all of which warrant being considered normal. Much is homeostatic. Much is the joy of humanity; some is its sorrow.

Understanding neurophysiologic constructs is one of science's great frontiers. Important insights have been forthcoming as to basic mechanisms. Clinical investigation is stymied by the bluntness of the available methodology and also by the need to define a referent population, one that is either "normal" or distinctive. The literature that relates to "fibromyalgia" is illustrative in this regard.

As stated above, patients with persistent widespread pain have a set of neurophysiologic constructs that supports their illness. They are living life under a pall and in such distress that they have sought care. In so doing, they have acquired counterproductive illness behaviors and a distinctive sick role. There must be special fine structures to their neurophysiologic constructs. Some will be shared by others who live life under a pall but do not experience persistent widespread pain, or if they do, they do not choose to be patients. Some of these people have plenty of "tender points" and probably share the "evidence for central sensitization" that patients labeled with fibromyalgia exhibit and share with others who have functional somatic syndromes.[39] Neither group likes to be poked or prodded. If one wants to probe the distinctiveness of the neurophysiologic construct that is labeled fibromyalgia, what is the proper comparison group? Certainly, randomly chosen "normal" people would be no more appropriate than selecting people of the blithest of spirits.

The results of clinical investigations probing the neuroscience and neuroendocrinology that associate with persistent widespread pain in patients who are labeled with fibromyalgia are inconsistent, irreproducible, subtle, or nonspecific. The latest assault on the secrets of the biology of fibromyalgia recruited cerebral functional imaging techniques. Alterations in cerebral blood flow and "activation" have been detected. Time will tell if these differences are reproducible. Science will tell if they are meaningful. Epidemiology will tell if they speak to more than the fact that patients found to have fibromyalgia have a distinctive neurophysiologic construct. The pharmaceutical industry is not put off by such uncertainty, particularly when the potential market is considerable. The Food and Drug Administration now accepts fibromyalgia as a therapeutic target and has licensed three drugs aimed at the putatively distinctive neurophysiologic construct. Two are already licensed as antidepressants; one is used for nerve damage in diabetes. All have exceedingly marginal benefits for patients labeled with fibromyalgia and even more marginal benefit-risk ratios.[40] All are selling briskly.

Could it be that there are no qualitatively distinctive markers? Could it be that the analysis of the biology of medically inexplicable persistent widespread pain will have to wait for the technology that will allow for the dissection of the fine structure of neurophysiologic constructs and the epidemiology that can cope with individual differences? Obviously, this is my conclusion. Fibromyalgia is a bad idea accepted and harbored by people who need to learn to substitute a better idea.[41] I would argue that any such label promotes a circularity of reasoning; it forces one to prove or disprove the entity rather than explore the concept. Furthermore, the label evokes a course of action that is unsupported by a demonstration of benefit, and it is ripe with unintended consequences, such as the vortex of disability determination that will occupy us later.

There is a counterargument. Specific labeling, such as fibromyalgia, establishes identity and community, targets the training of health-care providers, provides research criteria, facilitates communication (gives everyone something to Google), and facilitates indemnification. The debate is an exercise in value pluralism. My position is bolstered by the sad fate of so many despite their labels.[42]

Suffering and the Health of the Public

Some 10 percent of people spend every day coping with widespread pain, of which back pain is a prominent component. Most have more challenges in their lives, all sorts of financial and personal stresses. There are others, probably more in number, with these stresses who cope or try to cope in a fashion that does not need to accommodate physical symptoms. There are too many in our community who know not much in the way of joie d'vivre. Others walk too fine a line between satisfaction and despair. These people live, or can live, lives that are less pleasant and less lengthy.[43] They should be a great concern of any public-health agenda.

Much of this is a matter for the body politic. As I will argue in the chapters that follow, much of the suffering from chronic pain relates to economics and job satisfaction, but not all. Some reflects a style of coping that is learned in childhood.[44] It is not the pain that drives sufferers to seek medical care; it is the suffering consequent to the uncertainties that the pain precipitates in their mind. It is suffering that is their chief complaint. It is suffering that demands recognition and care.

FOUR

Doc, My Back Is Killing Me

In surveys of primary-care practices in many countries, pain is the most frequent, or nearly most frequent, complaint that causes a person with a predicament to become a patient with an illness. Furthermore, musculoskeletal pain is by far the most frequent pain complaint, and the low back is first among the body parts involved.[1] Given the ubiquity of low back pain in community surveys, it follows that only a fraction of those who suffer low back pain choose to become patients, and of those who so choose, not all will seek care for the next episode of pain. It is reasonable to assume that those who choose to become patients do so because their low back pain is particularly severe, so severe that they seek medical advice. That may seem the most sensible explanation, but it is wrong. We have known it to be wrong for forty years at least.

The classic study by Jiri Horal is illustrative.[2] In Sweden's national health-insurance scheme, the physician sick-lists a patient who is temporarily incapacitated for work. Horal randomly selected 212 of all the people in Gothenburg who were sick-listed by their general practitioners for low back pain in the previous year. From those sick-listed for something other than backache, he chose 212 matched for gender, age, and socioeconomic status with the 212 backache patients. He then went into the community to examine and X-ray all 424 patients (Table 4). It is no surprise that all of the patients who were sick-listed for backache in the previous year recalled the episode. The surprise is that nearly two-thirds of those sick-listed for something other than backache also recalled backache in the previous year. Furthermore, there was no clinical feature that distinguished the backache of those who had complained of backache from those who did not complain. Neither the quality of the backache, nor the physical examination,

TABLE 4. Comparison of Primary-Care Patients Who Had Sought Care for Low Back Pain in the Prior Year and Those without Low Back Pain in Horal's Gothenburg Survey

	PATIENTS WITH LOW BACK PAIN	PATIENTS WITHOUT LOW BACK PAIN
Total subjects	212	212
Recalled backache in the prior year	100%	67%
Recalled recurring backache	90%	68%
Recalled persistent backache	32%	31%
Radiographic disc disease	46%	32%
Older than 60	58%	60%

Source: J. Horal, "The Clinical Appearance of Low Back Disorders in the City of Gothenburg, Sweden: Comparisons of Incapacitated Probands with Matched Controls," Acta Orthopaedica Scandinavica 118, suppl. (1969): 1–109.

nor the radiographs were distinctive. Something else had to be at work in determining who would complain of backache and who would not.

One of the greatest accomplishments of clinical investigation in the twentieth century is the understanding of the "something else." If all patients and physicians could be brought up to speed, so many patients would be better served. However, we are imbued with Sydenham's disease-illness paradigm (chapter 3), so imbued that we will go to lengths to find the pathoanatomical cause of our regional back pain with the hope that it can be brought to heel in some biochemical or surgical triumph. My goal in this chapter is to commence the discussion of the "something else" that will carry over into subsequent chapters. But first I need to demonstrate the futility of the disease-illness paradigm in the setting of regional back pain.

Acute versus Chronic Regional Back Pain

Acute regional low back pain is quite different from chronic regional low back pain. Acute low back pain comes on suddenly[3] and hurts in relation to activity.[4] Chronic low back pain takes on a life of its own—a life that is more pained than it is painful. Chronic low back pain is far less related to activities, less localized to the low back itself, and usually accompanied by other somatic and affective symptoms.[5] "Chronic" does not refer to how long something lasts. Chronic regional low back pain denotes a condition wherein the suffering experienced in the setting of low back pain overwhelms the painfulness of the low back. In this chapter, we will focus on acute low back pain. Chapter 8 focuses on chronic low back pain and the disabilities with which it is always associated.

The Disease That Causes Acute Regional Low Back Pain

Many people have put forth theories of the cause of regional low back pain. These theories run the gamut from the fatuous and metaphysical to the putatively scientific. Yet theories are merely hypotheses yet to be disproved. No one should assume anything else. That is not the way of the world, however. The theory that is supported by authority is likely to emerge as the truth of the moment.

This has been termed "eminence-based medicine," and it has always raised my hackles. A "theory" is an assertion of uncertainty. If it is the best we can do, so be it. But let's not leap to the conclusion that because it is the best we can do, it is truth. Since my years in medical school, I have been composing aphorisms about medicine as I see it, which I call the "Laws of Therapeutic Dynamics."[6] The second law is: "There has never been a quack without a theory."

It is the legacy of Sydenham that there must be a disease, or more particularly an instance of pathoanatomy, that underlies low back pain. And indeed there must be. There is no guarantee, however, that we can identify the disease or that, if we could, whether we could do something for the patient. In the case of low back pain, finding diseases in the spine is not the issue. The challenge is discerning which, if any, of the prevalent spine diseases is causing the hurt today. Our spines were last "normal" and pristine when we were teenagers. If you have a pristine spine at age sixty, it is quite "abnormal." By forty, nearly all of us have acquired impressive changes in the anatomy of our spines. Many will have osteophytes ("spurs") around one or more of the three joints that make up each vertebral level of the lumbosacral spine. Nearly all will have changes in one or more discs, the joints that attach one vertebral body directly to another. Since nearly all of us have these changes whether we are hurting or not, the challenge is not to find a change but to find *the* change that is associated with the hurting. That's a lesson that has been hard learned, and it remains hard to teach today—even to the medical community.

I am about to argue that the imaging studies of the spine in patients who have acute (or chronic) regional low back pain are irrelevant at best and misleading all too often. Given the compelling science that supports this assertion, I feel no need to teach the anatomy of the spine. However, all the patients of all sorts of practitioners are likely to be bombarded with anatomical terminology of varying sophistication. Many will have the images of their spine laid before their horrified eyes. Since these experiences can overwhelm reason, a brief explanation of the anatomy of the lumbosacral spine should forearm any listener. Hence, I have provided Figures 2 and 3, each with a lengthy explicatory caption. For generations, physicians have touted radiographs and, more recently, far more exacting imaging studies as holding the secret to the cause of backache. That may be true, but no one has unlocked that secret for regional back pain, and assertions to the contrary regarding sciatica are hardly more convincing.

Imaging the Spine

Why do physicians feel compelled to order X-rays to define the anatomy of the lumbosacral spines of patients with regional low back pain? Health agencies in eleven countries have published evidence-based guidelines for the management of such patients; all agree that radiographs are not useful.[7] Almost everything one can see on an X-ray is likely to be present in many people the same age who are not hurting, is likely to have been present before the current episode of backache, and is likely to persist after the episode. The only changes one might find that could correlate with the episode is a straightening of the lumbar curve, but that, too, is a common finding as we age and can be seen by simply looking at the patient's back.

Why do we submit to such studies, even expect them? Many years ago in a study in the military, soldiers reporting to sick call for low back pain were randomized to receive X-rays or not. Of course, whether they got the X-rays or not made no difference in treatment prescribed or clinical outcome. However, many of the soldiers who were not X-rayed went to a provider off the base and got themselves X-rayed. We have been taught that the choice to be a patient with low back pain is a choice to seek a cause and a cure. X-rays are part of this preconception, even if the images are irrelevant. Preconceptions die hard.

We live in a culture that is enamored of technological advances. The industry that is committed to imaging the spine is enormous and enormously profitable. Computerized tomography (CT) scanners and magnetic-resonance-imaging (MRI) machines are cash cows for their manufacturers,

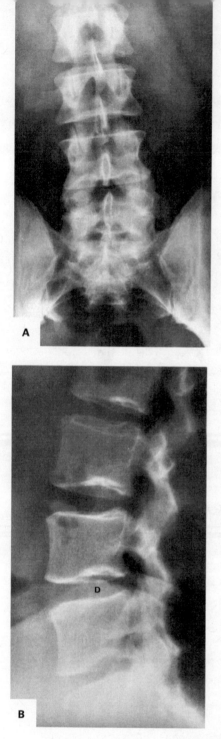

FIGURE 2. The spine is a series of bones called the vertebrae. In the center of the vertebrae is the spinal canal, through which runs the spinal cord and the nerve roots as they exit the spinal cord. Each vertebra has three components: the posterior elements form the roof of the canal, the vertebral body is the floor, and the pedicles connect them on either side. The spinal canal is formed by the alignment of these vertebral elements. The alignment is maintained by the articulation of the posterior elements and strong fibrous tissues elsewhere. The radiographs shown here are of a pretty normal lumbar spine. Radiographs are like a photograph, but they use X-rays instead of light to expose the film (or the detector, since most X-rays are now digitized similar to a digital camera). The efficiency with which X-rays penetrate through the body depends on the type of tissue they encounter; the denser the tissue, the less they can pass through and the more the image appears white. Well-mineralized, dense bone blocks X-rays and appears white, whereas air containing tissues appear black. Shades of gray speak to the varying density of the tissues.

In Frame A, the view is as if you were looking through the belly at the spine; Frame B is the view from the side. In Frame A, the vertebral bodies are the rectangular shadows that seem to be floating. The dense elliptical structures in the midline are the spinous processes that protrude from the center of the posterior elements; these are the bumps we can feel with our fingers in the middle of our backs. In Frame B, the vertebral bodies appear squarer and can be seen to be attached by bone to the posterior elements. The space between the vertebral bodies appears empty and black, but it is anything but empty. The vertebral bodies are connected by a complex soft tissue called the disc (I have placed a *D* in one of the disc "spaces").

As mentioned, this is a relatively pristine spine. As we age, discal tissue changes in composition, disc spaces narrow, and degenerative changes become commonplace in the vertebral bodies and the posterior elements. These changes lead to increased bone density and the development of bone spurs.

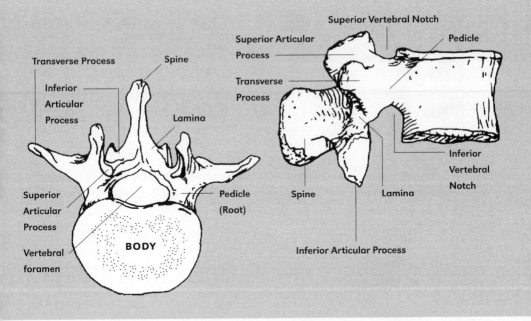

FIGURE 3. These diagrams offer some of the anatomical detail that correlates with the description of the structures apparent in the radiographs in Figure 2. The perspective in the upper diagram is looking down the spine at a vertebra. The spinal canal (vertebral foramen) is obvious, as are the structures that delineate this space. The vertebral bodies and the intervertebral discs are the floor, the pedicles are the walls, and the posterior elements are the roof. The parts of the roof that are closest to the spinal cord are the lamina, which are the target of the laminectomies performed by surgeons who will earn my disdain in chapter 6 for doing such violence to this structure.

The lower diagram correlates with the radiograph in Frame B of Figure 2, the side view. You can see the spine of the vertebra protruding back from the posterior elements. You can also see structures in the posterior elements protruding up, toward the head, and down. They are the superior and inferior articular processes, respectively. In the articulated spine, they are juxtaposed to the articular processes of the neighboring vertebrae to form joints that allow motion and contribute to the stability of the spinal column. These joints are called "facet joints." None of us are spared degenerative changes in facet joints as we age.

With articulation, the inferior vertebral notch of one vertebra is opposed to the superior vertebral notch of the vertebra below, forming a foramen (hole) through which nerves exit the spinal canal. One can see that the nerve would course over the disc at that level.

the institutions that house them, and the people who operate them. The trouble with medical technological advances is that we cannot evaluate the degree to which we are benefited. If you purchase a car with a GPS or a DVD player or some other gizmo, you have yourself to blame if you discover you have no need that justifies the added expense. If you are paying an insurance premium that is inflated to share the cost of imaging the spines of people with regional back pain, you have no way to know if the money is well spent.

"Low specificity" limits the diagnostic utility of CT and MRI scans as much as it limits that of radiographs. "Low specificity" means that we can define anatomy but not discern anatomy that is specific to today's regional backache. That is no surprise. As we said, mature spines are likely to exhibit many pathologic changes. MRI scans are brilliant at defining the details of the soft tissues and CT scans of the bony anatomy. Imaging has a high false-positive rate, with the result that billions of dollars are spent annually in this pointless exercise. Furthermore, magnetic resonance imaging cannot be used to predict back pain.[8] Magnetic resonance imaging is not even sensitive to anatomical changes that might correlate with new symptoms.[9] Cost has little to do with cost-effectiveness if imaging is ineffective.

To be fair, many physicians and most radiologists are aware of this. Few are willing to declare that degenerative changes are normal, as I am. But few are willing to declare that degenerative change is the cause of the problem. Nonetheless, savvy physicians order these imaging studies, and savvy radiologists are all too willing to provide them. This may reflect their concern that, while the scientific studies pertain to most patients, they may not pertain to a particular patient's problem.[10]

Such a hit-and-miss rationale aside, imaging the spine has been the first resort of medical practitioners and the expectation of their patients for generations. Imaging might not facilitate return to well-being, but it certainly contributes to patient satisfaction.[11] Is this a valuable outcome? Or is this sense of satisfaction contributing to the persistence of illness? The patient-physician discourse that follows imaging always relates to the demonstrable pathoanatomy. That discourse may be satisfying, but it is associated with an exacerbation of pain.[12] If the image discussed is generated by MRI, the discourse is also associated with an increased likelihood of surgery.[13]

Imaging is not serving as a diagnostic tool in this setting. It is one element of a complex treatment drama that endows patients with unfounded notions of pathophysiology and enriches their narrative of distress with the private vocabulary of the treating professional. Patients are forever changed by these experiences, too few for the better.[14] Whatever "satisfaction" is derived from undergoing imaging studies does not stop a third of primary-care patients with back pain from using multiple practitioners.[15] In this context, imaging is symbolic of the flawed logic that contributes to the myths about back pain that are so prevalent in the community and renders the prognosis for the return to a sense of well-being so dismal.[16]

On the Wear-and-Tear Fallacy

Who among us can look at an image of our own spine and not feel disquiet as we come to realize how many discs have degenerated, how many facet joints have spurs, how peculiar is the alignment? What has gone wrong? What will happen to me? What did I do? What should I avoid? Given the common horror of disease, these queries and the accompanying angst are predictable. We all need to be disabused.

Research over the past decade informs all of these questions. The timing and the degree to which our spines acquire these changes have almost nothing to do with what we do or do not do in life. Heredity has the dominant role, accounting for as much as 75 percent of the variance.[17] Pattern of usage through life has a barely discernible influence. The notion of "wear and tear" needs to be discarded. This paradigm shift has major implications for policy in the context of workplace health and safety.

The ramifications are far-reaching. The predominant role of genetics in the magnitude of degenerative changes at the spine, coupled with the fact that these changes do not correlate with clinical events such as back pain, calls for a dramatic shift in the common sense regarding regional backache. Not only is spinal pathology genetically predestined, but the genetic predisposition for degenerative changes in the hands, spine, and knees also renders these processes among the most heritable of polygenic traits. They are far more heritable than almost all of the other traits we hear so much about in the medical press, far more than cardiovascular disease, cancer, dementia, and longevity. Furthermore, these spinal degenerative changes have almost no association with illness: a person who displays a great deal of degenerative change is no more likely to have back pain than one who does not.

Degenerative disease of the spine is a genetically driven concomitant of aging, like graying or balding. We need to "get over it."

Evidence-Based Treatment of Regional Low Back Pain

In chapter 3, I suggested that one of the great accomplishments of modern epidemiology was the development of the methodology for testing the effectiveness of treatments. When my generation entered medicine, such scholarship was a cottage industry—but not for long. The Cochrane Collaboration (⟨www.cochrane.org⟩) pioneered the institutionalization of the exercise of critically examining the literature and drawing inferences as to the quality of the evidence.[18] The gold standard for evidence is the randomized controlled trial (RCT). The underlying principle is straightforward: one randomly assigns half the sample of patients who are candidates for the treatment into a group that is treated and the other half into a group that is not treated (the control group) and then determines if there is a difference in outcome between the groups. Careers of statisticians and epidemiologists have been committed to the fine-tuning of this methodology. The Cochrane Collaboration's mission is to identify those interventions for which there is evidence of efficacy. Topics are chosen for review, and the relevant literature is systematically searched out and then analyzed as to quality by predefined criteria. The format is highly structured and the criteria for the systematic review so rigorous that typically only a few high-quality articles, nearly always RCTs, are identified among the many for any given topic. The group then sets to the task of drawing some conclusions as to whether evidence has emerged and to what degree it is compelling on methodological grounds. This is termed the "level of evidence."

The mission of the Cochrane Collaboration stops short of judgments as to whether the magnitude of the effect is sufficient to justify doing the intervention to a patient. Few of the organizations involved in establishing the evidentiary basis for clinical practices take on the assessment of clinical relevance. The American College of Physicians' Journal Club takes papers one at a time, makes a determination of the robustness of the evidence, and offers some assessment of clinical efficacy or lack thereof. But most shy away from such conclusions for reasons that have never been clear to me. Establishing criteria for a meaningful "level of effectiveness" is a more demanding challenge than establishing criteria for a meaningful "level of evidence." Nonetheless, when there is evidence for an effect, "is it an important effect?" is the crucial next query.

The Cochrane Collaboration is named for Archibald Cochrane, who emerged from medically ministering to his fellow prisoners of war in

Germany in World War II with the burning need to define clinical efficacy. He studied epidemiology at the foot of Bradford Hill, one of the founding fathers of modern epidemiology—the epidemiology of workplace health and safety in particular. Cochrane commenced his academic career in Cardiff. In 1972 he called for analyzing randomized clinical trials as the most scientific way to inform the practice of medicine. The cause was taken up by thought leaders at McMaster University in Canada (notably Brian Haynes and David Sackett) and Yale (Alvan Feinstein in particular). In 1993 these and some seventy other researchers announced the formation of the Cochrane Collaboration "to prepare, maintain, and disseminate systematic reviews of the effects of health care interventions."* In 2003 it was estimated that some 10,000 reviews are necessary to provide a comprehensive "evidence-based medicine" library with periodic updating of all reviews.[19] That is an underestimate. There is much work to do, particularly since the available 4,000 reviews (and probably the available RCTs) do not reflect the global burden of disease.[20]

The "Back Review Group" has produced many reviews in the decade since it was established.[21] It has gone to some effort to hone the criteria by which it rates the available literature and draws conclusions as to the presence of evidence and its quality.[22] This is neither a trivial exercise nor one with firm rules. Applying different criteria for "level of evidence" leads to quite different conclusions in Cochrane reviews of interventions for low back pain.[23] While it is not the only source of reviews seeking evidence for or against interventions for low back pain or other disorders, the Cochrane Collaboration remains the leader in this exercise because of its methodological rigor,[24] though time will tell if this approach is prescient. But we do not have to wait to demonstrate that when you compare Cochrane reviews with industry-supported meta-analyses of the same agent, the industry-sponsored reviewers choose methodological approaches that are far more likely to support a conclusion favorable to the sponsor's product.[25]

*Today the collaboration is made up of fifty-one Collaborative Review Groups, thirteen Methods Groups, and sixteen Field/Network Groups with about 14,000 reviewers in over ninety countries. These are orchestrated by twenty-six Coordinating Centers dispersed across thirteen countries. An elected steering group oversees the entire effort supported by a secretariat based in Oxford, United Kingdom. Most of the participants are volunteering their time. The entire undertaking survives on meager contributions from many countries. To date, the Cochrane Collaboration has shunned support from pharmaceutical firms and the like, although individual reviewers are not restricted in that regard.

The Cochrane Back Review Group is performing a valuable service, but not the service one might guess. Given the compulsive nature of their literature review, they can provide reassurance to those of us who review the literature on our own that we have missed nothing of importance. For example, I have no interest in prescribing "muscle relaxants." First, I don't think the data support any effect on muscles from these drugs. Second, all they offer is grogginess, which I find a poor way to take the edge off of low back pain. The Cochrane Back Group came to the same conclusion based on thirty trials, most of which were considered high quality.[26] The literature on insoles is scant and not at all compelling.[27] There is no hint of benefiting from all kinds of traction in twenty-five RCTs, five deemed high in quality.[28] Traction is in the archives. As for applying heat or cold to the back, the evidence is limited and unimpressive.[29] That I will leave up to the patient. But bed rest deserves an extensive evidence-based discussion. No one should be told to go to bed for a backache. The evidence-based advice is to get on with life as best you can.

You get the idea. There are thousands of trials probing the efficacy of the items on the therapeutic menu for acute regional low back pain. These trials are all attempts to test the efficacy of a particular "modality," a pill or poke or gizmo, on the course of a patient who is entangled in a complex treatment act of which the modality is only one element. In all these trials, the control groups fare pretty well. With the exception of nonsteroidal anti-inflammatory drugs, no modality that is traditionally under the purview of a physician can be shown to improve on the rate of healing or on the intensity of the pain during healing over that seen in the control patients. Thus speaks the evidence.

We need not abandon the treatment act, just the hocus-pocus of nearly all the treatment modalities. But we need to make sure the treatment act itself is palliative in the short and long term. That is not a simple agenda given all the individual differences in patients and physicians. Some of the secret to palliation may be forthcoming from an appreciation of the psychosocial confounders to coping with which we will come to grips shortly.

Guidelines for the Treatment of Low Back Pain

It is not clear how efficiently "level of evidence" translates into the quality of care in practice. The impact on clinical practice probably depends more on word of mouth and physician networking than any formalized continuing education.[30] No one likes to have his or her preconceived notions and comfortable practices challenged, not even physicians. One response to the uneven understanding of the evidentiary basis of medicine is the formulation of treatment guidelines based on the evidence.

As mentioned above, many countries have produced guidelines for the treatment of regional back pain. Some, notably New Zealand, have pioneered the notion of "yellow flags," which are clues in the patient's history to psychosocial challenges that may be confounding the patient's course. Most, however, are the work of committees performing analyses similar to those undertaken by the Cochrane Collaboration and then basing the recommendations in their guidelines on those analyses. The guidelines are predictably similar across countries. None recommends surgery or other invasive procedures for acute regional low back pain. Two of these exercises are worthy of special attention because they set the precedents for the guidelines that are in use today and are object lessons in the politics of writing such a document. A third set of guidelines is hot off the press and worth a look as state of the art.

Report of the Quebec Task Force on Spinal Disorders

In 1983 the Quebec Workers' Health and Safety Commission was faced with underwriting a dramatic escalation in physiotherapy treatments for workers with disabling regional back pain, so-called back injuries. They commissioned the Institute for Workers' Health and Safety to undertake an analysis of the appropriate management of such injuries. A task force was assembled, chaired by Walter O. Spitzer, a renowned epidemiologist on the McGill University faculty. The charge was to "develop and test a typology for the various treatments," create "matrices for the evaluation of both diagnostic and therapeutic measures," and "make recommendations designed to improve the quality of treatment for injured workers with these morbid conditions of the spine."

Spitzer assembled a group that was divided equally among clinicians, allied health professionals, and methodologists and somehow managed to drive a consensus that appeared as a report in *Spine* in 1987.[31] The methodology was pioneering and set the precedent for the Cochrane Collaboration and many to follow. For example, papers that were anecdotal, observational, or derivative carried no weight, whereas RCTs were considered the gold standard.

The task force also set the precedent for controversy in an exercise such as this. For example, many treatments were supported only by anecdote and conviction, and these, even if in "common practice," would be denoted as not supported by scientific evidence. That designation is not the same as "CONTRAINDICATED on the basis of scientific evidence," but it is damning nonetheless and pulled the rug out from under a number of professions that based their professionalism on untested remedies. Representatives of these professions distanced themselves from the task force and its report, and so little came of the exercise in terms of policy.

Clinical Practice Guideline Number 14

The Agency for Health Care Policy and Research (AHCPR) was created by the Omnibus Budget Reconciliation Act of 1989 during the George H. W. Bush administration and commissioned to develop guidelines to standardize the evaluation and treatment of conditions with high prevalence, morbidity, mortality, cost, and variability of practice style. The legislation was passed despite vigorous, even strident debate by nearly all stakeholders—including the American Medical Association—all decrying a philosophy that imposed population-based health care on individual choice. Nonetheless, the AHCPR set to its task, producing documents relating to the management of postoperative pain, incontinence in the elderly, pressure ulcers, and more. Each document was met with controversy of varying degree, usually as to the comprehensiveness and generalizability of the inferences based on available RCTs. After all, the RCTs of the highest quality tend to randomize a highly selected group of patients, so that the results might not generalize to patients with the same disorder but with other clinical attributes.

The controversy reached a fever pitch with Number 14, the Clinical Practice Guideline for Acute Low Back Problems in Adults.[32] Number 14 was the product of a panel chaired by Stanley Bigos, an orthopedist, and composed of twenty-two clinicians of assorted ilk and one consumer advocate. I am very familiar with this panel, its process, its product, and the aftermath, as I served as one of three official consultants to the panel. The process essentially followed the model of the Quebec task force, but with more recent literature. Over 10,000 published studies were considered. Nonetheless, they reached quite similar conclusions, pointing out that much that was common practice had no scientific support, and some was contraindicated. In particular, physical modalities, invasive procedures, and imaging suffered mightily.

Thanks to the Quebec precedent, no stakeholder was caught unaware.

The backlash was far more concerted to say the least, and it was often vitriolic. The physiatrists produced a rebuttal in book form,[33] arguing that since all too often there was no good evidence one way or the other, why not trust clinical judgment? The spine surgical community produced attacks on many fronts. The North American Spine Society, the professional organization for practicing spine surgeons, convened its own panel, which revisited the same literature but reached quite different conclusions.

The spine surgeons found a more direct path for redress for what they perceived as a biased exercise perpetrated by the AHCPR: they commenced a campaign aimed at Congress. With the support of the surgeons, the Center for Patient Advocacy came into existence and lobbied Congress vigorously against the AHCPR at a time when majority leader Newt Gingrich was calling for reductions in the size and influence of the federal government. In 1995 the AHCPR was eliminated as a wasteful government agency. It was to rise again, but only as a shadow of its former self, as the Agency for Healthcare Research and Quality, a data "clearinghouse" that no longer was to draw conclusions meant to constrain clinical practice. The British government created the National Institute for Health and Clinical Excellence (NICE), a body similar to the AHCPR, to create practice guidelines based on evidence. It is not clear whether NICE is any more effective at influencing physician practices.[34]

Although government supported, the Cochrane Collaboration and NICE have a conflict-of-interest taint by virtue of the commercial activities of some of their participating experts. This is not unusual. In a survey of more than 200 practice guidelines from around the world, more than a third of the experts on the panels had ties to relevant drug companies and more than 70 percent of panels were affected.[35] I find this highly distressing, and so do others, with good reason. Conflict of interest should exclude "experts" from panels and editorial authorships simply because self-interest, subliminal or not, cannot be weighed by those who are to be influenced. This is an argument to which I will return.

The American College of Physicians and the American Pain Society

Guidelines were also produced by the American College of Physicians (ACP) and the American Pain Society (APS).[36] The exercise is familiar. The system for grading the literature is similar. The essence of the guidelines that emerged and the basis for the recommendations are summarized in Table 5. Much of importance is in the details, and much of importance is

TABLE 5. Guidelines Generated by the American College of Physicians and the American Pain Society for Regional Low Back Pain

RECOMMENDATION	STRENGTH OF RECOMMENDATION	QUALITY OF EVIDENCE
Assess psychosocial risk factors for chronicity	Strong	Moderate
Do not image the spine routinely	Strong	Moderate
Only image the spine for systemic disease or neurological compromise	Strong	Moderate
Advise patients as to prognosis	Strong	Moderate
Advise patients to stay active	Strong	Moderate
Prescribe only acetaminophen or NSAIDS* for analgesia	Strong	Moderate
If patients are not improving, consider nonpharmacologic therapy	Weak	Moderate

Source: R. Chou, A. Qaseem, V. Snow, and others, "Diagnosis and Treatment of Low Back Pain: A Joint Clinical Practice Guideline for the American College of Physicians and the American Pain Society," Annals of Internal Medicine 147 (2007): 478–91.

Note: The guidelines are broader, encompassing other presentations, but this table focuses on regional back pain.

*Nonsteroidal anti-inflammatory drugs

glossed over. For example, there are psychosocial risk factors for chronicity, but we will discover later that our ability to sort them out is limited, our ability to find the leading issue is even more limited, and our ability to do something about them is arguable. Furthermore, much that is useless is captured by the notion of "nonpharmacologic therapies" (mainly physical modalities such as traction); what is useful is barely so. Hence the recommendation is weak and pertains only to the particular treatments and not to the treatment regimens of which they are a part. Therapies that are recommended based on the evidence have some effectiveness, but this is not predictable and is seldom dramatic. The evidence does not speak to effectiveness in this fashion, and like other guidelines, neither does the ACP/APS document.

The upshot is that there is no reason to seek medical care for a regional backache, certainly no reason that responds to Sydenham's disease-illness paradigm. The only possible justification would be that your physician can provide a port in the storm: empathy, wisdom, reassurance, and constructive advice. There is no magic hiding in the black bag, and there is probably no black bag either. The same pertains to any other port one might choose in this storm. No one has a better bag of tricks.

These are hard-won insights, and they seem counterintuitive in our medicalized world. The fact is that you may be best off if you do not tell anyone about your regional backache and try to get on with it. Once you complain, you become a patient in a treatment act that is informed by these ACP/APS guidelines but not strongly compelled by them. Do you have an "acute" backache, or have your symptoms gone on longer than four weeks? Do you have a regional backache, or is there some neurological complication? These are judgments, and if they are affirmative, the ACP/APS guidelines will be superseded by literature that considers other questions. In particular, invasive options by needle and knife will come to the fore. The ACP/APS guidelines only give this eventuality brief lip service.

The Reasons for Choosing to Be a Patient

Coping with regional back pain is always a challenge and involves several key considerations. There is the personal effect to process: How and how much is function restricted? How and how much is comfort compromised? What vocational and personal activities are compromised or precluded? There are the options to consider: Is the back pain bearable? Do symptoms require use of any of the myriad pharmaceuticals (agents, unctions, and potions) and devices that have been widely purveyed and forcefully marketed to prejudice the decision? Is professional assistance needed in coping? The roster of professionals who will provide assistance, for a fee, is considerable. How do patients choose between purveyors?

The conventional wisdom is that the decision to seek treatment is driven by the physical intensity of the predicament. The more severe the pain, the more likely that it will be memorable, will result in the use of analgesics, will render one unable to work, and will lead to seeking professional health care. Epidemiology has put this common wisdom to the test, and it is no longer tenable. The common denominator that drives the decision making is a compromise in one's ability to cope.[37] Workplace-based[38] and community-based[39] cohort studies have probed associations with the recall and reporting of lower back pain as well as arm and knee pain. Psychological distress at home or at work, aspects of illness behaviors, and other somatic symptoms also are important. Furthermore, psychosocial confounders to coping are as important in rendering the back pain persistent as they are in rendering the pain reportable in the first place.[40]

This insight has great implications for clinical treatment, whether or not it is orchestrated by a medical practitioner. The narrative of distress of a patient with regional back pain should be probed as a surrogate complaint.[41] "My back hurts" is likely to mean, "My back hurts but I'm really here because I can't cope with this episode right now."[42] However, for three centuries physicians, nearly all other health-care professionals, and society at large have not been able to conceptualize "my back hurts" in this fashion. The possibility that back pain is but one's last straw is counterintuitive, and the suggestion can be anathema to the patient, tantamount to saying "it's in your mind." The acceptable notion is that back pain is simply the manifestation of an important underlying disease, just as coughing purulent sputum is a manifestation of bacterial pneumonia. Any reduction in one's ability to cope is assumed to be a consequence of back pain, not the reason back pain is less tolerable. *Disease* is the culprit that must be palliated if it cannot be expunged.

All health-care professionals have theories of the cause of the problem on which they base their therapeutic approach. Most theories hold that something in or about the back has gone terribly wrong. For regional back pain, though, no theory has stood up to scientific testing. As for the various treatment regimens and interventions—the modalities—none has proven a match for regional back pain and very few have any demonstrable effectiveness. Rather than question the premise, clinicians and patients are wont to cast about for different theories and approaches. Imaging only serves to bolster the notion that back pain is nothing more than the symptom of an underlying disease. This social construct does more to sustain an enormous treatment enterprise than it does to help the patient.

Individuals with regional backache might fare less poorly by managing as best they can,[43] perhaps with some lay advice,[44] than by choosing to become patients. If the statement "I can't cope with this backache" were the customary complaint when patients sought care, perhaps they would fare better.[45] Today, medicine does not seem able to breach the disease-illness divide[46] or develop the skills to apply these insights.[47]

FIVE

The Quest for a Better Way; Or,
My Name Is Nortin and I'm a Placebo?

As we concluded in the previous chapter, medicine has no simple cure for regional low back pain. Neither does medicine own the exclusive right to try to find one, nor has it ever. In antiquity, gods and demigods could cause and cure diseases and wounds. The Greek demigod Asclepios, a son of Apollo, begot two sons, Machaon the surgeon and Podalirios the physician, and two daughters, Hygieia and Panacea. These healing gods were enshrined in special temples open to all who were ill and suffering. Physicians were itinerant craftsmen ministering in the homes of those who could pay their fee.

It fell to Hippocrates to confront all this mythology. Hippocrates was born on the island of Cos about 460 BCE. On his death at the age of eighty, he left a legacy of shrewd clinical observations and ethical commentaries meant to extricate medicine from the morass of metaphysics. Influenced by his contemporary Plato, Hippocrates cast aside precedent, theosophical notions, and superstitions to found the "dogmatist" school of medicine. For the dogmatists, observation was a poor substitute for reasoning. To Hippocrates' way of thinking, the health of the body depended on vital forces. Vitalistic theories led to therapeutic measures such as purging, bleeding, and dehydrating the ill.

The history of medicine ever since has involved the discarding of vitalistic theories in favor of those that are scientifically tenable and the fashioning of remedies that temper therapeutic zeal with requirements for evidence of effectiveness. This process was hardly linear, however. There were infrequent conceptual leaps: Harvey's notion of circulation and Sydenham's disease-illness paradigm, for example. There was the occasional therapeutic leap: Joseph Lister's antisepsis, Edward Jenner's vaccination, and William T. G. Morton's anesthesia. But most of medicine remained vitalism dressed in the scientific jargon of the day well into the twentieth century, and most of what passed as therapeutics was based on these pseudoscientific inferences and often was toxic if not brutal.

Many in the United States and many more around the globe still seek refuge in various forms of metaphysics, superstition, and theology when they are not well, sometimes by default and sometimes with good reason. After all, despite all the medical progress, to this day much of illness eludes scientific probing. Furthermore, the treatments of modern medicine are likely to be more painful, even more damaging, than whatever regimens alternative medicine supports. When the competition to salve the illness is between different schools of dogmatism (and that includes both medical and alternative treatment), the consumer should feel freer to choose or avoid them all.

Religion always offered a gentler alternative. Some religious movements are bolstered by a passive, faith-based approach to healing. The Pentecostal movement and Christian Science have been on the American scene for over a century; Scientology is a newcomer. Medicine had little advantage in the competition for the allegiance of the ill and hurting until the last half of the twentieth century, when scientific medicine finally had in its arsenal antibiotics, antihypertensives, diuretics, sophisticated surgery, and more. Medicine has achieved so much in the past fifty years that it merits and commands a perch atop the contemporary pecking order of healers. Today, it is egregious malpractice if a physician does not treat bacterial meningitis appropriately; it is also manslaughter if someone with bacterial meningitis is knowingly afforded only faith-based therapy. Medicine has limitations, however, that must be recognized, or progress is stymied and professionalism becomes a sham. Hubris is no less intolerable today than it was in antiquity, and imperiousness is as inexcusable. For some in medicine, those are bitter pills. Regardless, it is the price of professionalism.

Today, as has long been true, some remedies are beyond the reach of testing. Some are based on theories that defy academic reasoning and therefore earn the scorn of modern medical dogmatists. Take the example of *susto*. *Susto*, the Spanish word for "fright," is the folk diagnosis for the posttraumatic stress disorder (PTSD) that afflicts people indigenous to Peru and several other Latin American countries. It can be a pervasive, debilitating illness characterized by listlessness and other somatic complaints. Of all the folk remedies for *susto*, the most legendary is the *limpieza* or *barrida*, Spanish for "cleansing" and "sweeping," respectively. This quasi-religious, somewhat frenetic ritualistic ceremony is beyond the ken of most medical practitioners, who are likely to be disdainful of such a primitive and irrational form of psychotherapy.

Medical practitioners are more likely to prescribe psychotropic agents for PTSDs, even though these therapies have no basis in scientific evidence, according to a literature review undertaken by the Institute of Medicine (⟨www.iom.edu/CMS/3793/39330/47389.aspx⟩). The same review found evidence for exposure-based therapies such as "cognitive behavior therapy," which are as culturally constructed and linguistically determined as *limpieza*. While modern medicine is unlikely to countenance, let alone perform, frenetic rituals for *susto*, it is more than tolerant of medicalizing the PTSD that afflicts soldiers returning from battle or the driver whose neck pain persists after a rear-end motor vehicle accident in the absence of demonstrable anatomical damage. The latter is diagnosed as "whiplash" or "whiplash-associated disorders" (WAD), a notion with parallels to the experience of regional low back pain when it is conceptualized as an injury. "Whiplash-associated disorders" has superseded "whiplash" as the diagnosis, since more than neck pain can result from a minor rear-end motor vehicle accident. WAD can be a diffuse disorder with no identifiable physical cause that includes the syndrome of chronic widespread pain discussed in prior chapters.[1]

Whiplash-Associated Disorders

WAD hangs over the necks of drivers in the United States, Canada, Switzerland, and many other resource-advantaged countries like the sword of Damocles.[2] In these countries, a significant minority of people in a car that is struck (seldom is this the fate of occupants of the car that does the striking) suffer a prolonged and complex chronic pain state in the absence of demonstrable damage. The consequences of minor rear-end collisions are nearly always transient and self-limited in some other countries, including Lithuania, Greece,[3] and Germany.[4]

Some have argued that these differences reflected the differences in tort systems.[5] Swedes who choose not to pursue litigation following rear-end collisions, for example, suffer no long-term consequences compared to Swedes who sue regardless of the violence of the collision.[6] The "evil tort" argument was tenuous, however, until the recent analysis of the situation in Saskatchewan.[7] When Saskatchewan went to a no-fault system that eliminated awards for pain and suffering, the incidence of WAD plummeted with no demonstrable long-term health consequences for those involved in accidents.[8] The same is true in Saskatchewan for low back pain persisting after a minor accident.[9] Acute neck pain following a minor accident is in small part related to the violence of impact.[10] However, biomechanics has little if anything to do with the persistent neck pain or the other manifestations of WAD. Even rodeo athletes do not develop persistent neck pain, let alone WAD.[11] Furthermore, almost no patients experience persistent neck symptoms if they survive high-energy traffic accidents in which they sustain unrelated injuries requiring treatment.[12] WAD is socially constructed: the person susceptible to the notion can be led into a narrative of illness that is sustained by a particular treatment and insurance community that is committed to and profits from its continuation.

These ecological observations and natural experiments raise the specter, with some justification, of gain and even malfeasance on the part of the victims and the establishment that supports them. For me, there is no need to blame the victims. While most people who are the victims of rear-end motor vehicle accidents are aware of or made aware of WAD, and many are sore following the accident, only a few go on to experience WAD, even in the countries and jurisdictions where WAD supports a clinical, insurance, and legal industry. These unfortunate individuals are convinced that they have been seriously, even irreparably, harmed. Many find themselves in tort litigation seeking compensation for the horror of WAD, which they understand to have resulted from the biomechanical consequences of their accident.[13] Some learn to fear this outcome by virtue of being offered early aggressive care, which correlates with delayed recovery.[14] Most who are susceptible to such notions have preaccident depressive symptoms, passive coping styles,[15] and other psychosocial confounders.[16] Furthermore, many have an unshakable belief that WAD is their likely fate from the outset.[17]

The Cochrane Collaboration undertook a systematic review of the literature that bears on the treatments afforded patients with WAD.[18] According to the collaboration's findings, patients who have suffered no demonstrable tissue damage should avoid rest and collars and "maintain usual activities." Anything more than reassurance seems to predispose the susceptible minority to the fate they fear, with little hope that they can be brought back to some sense of feeling well ever again.[19]

WAD is an object lesson in socially constructing a disease by medicalizing a symptom that should seem surmountable to anyone free to reason independently. But WAD is not the only socially constructed disease where "healers" are ineffective at best and society seems too gullible to question the practices. A remarkable number of these socially constructed diseases relate to the regional musculoskeletal disorders, regional back pain in particular. WAD is notable for the magnitude of treatment-induced illness that can be mobilized in an "advantaged" medical system.

Placebo

A Peruvian with WAD might find some relief in *limpieza*. I doubt, though, that any native-born American would find *limpieza* an effective treatment, that any "modern" clinical setting would countenance the ritual, or that any insurer would indemnify it. We would consider it too "primitive" or "irrational" when compared to our iatrogenic (disease-inducing) "standard of care," which demands medical and physical interventions before some sort of psychological approach can be offered. Any benefit that might derive from *limpieza* would likely be dismissed as a placebo effect. In modern America, that is a condemnation. It is tantamount to accusing the sufferer of a flaw in character, either a psychological weakness or feigning. The implication that "it's in your mind" drives most to seek alternative theories of causation, upon which alternative treatments are based. Nearly always this involves the provision of a particular placebo by practitioners committed to its purveyance.

I do not use the term "placebo" to be contentious. There is no better alternative. There is a growing robust science probing the psychosocial components of a "placebo effect." For example, investigators in Boston recruited nearly 300 young adults from the community who had been experiencing regional musculoskeletal disorders of the arm for at least three months.[20] They were divided into two groups, each then randomized into a controlled trial for two months. In one trial, the subjects were subjected to acupuncture or sham acupuncture. In the other trial, the subjects were randomized to receive Amitriptyline or a placebo pill. In the acupuncture trial, all spent time twice weekly with an experienced acupuncturist who applied a sheathed needle to the skin repeatedly each session. For sham acupuncture, the procedure looks and feels the same, but the needle never pierces the skin. Everybody improved in both trials. However, the point of this exercise was not the separate trials but a comparison of the two

TABLE 6. Average Weekly Change (95 Percent Confidence Interval) in the Brigham Placebo Pill v. Placebo Acupuncture Comparison

	SHAM DEVICE	PLACEBO PILL	P VALUE
Pain (10-point scale)	−0.33 (−0.40 to −0.26)	−0.15 (−0.21 to −0.09)	<0.001
Grip strength (kg)	0.04 (−0.21 to +0.28)	0.05 (−0.15 to +0.24)	0.92

Source: J. Kaptchuk, W. B. Stason, R. B. Davis, A. T. R. Legedza, R. N. Schnyer, C. E. Kerr, D. A. Stone, B. H. Nam, I. Kirsch, and R. H. Goldman, "Sham Device v. Inert Pill: Randomised Controlled Trial of Two Placebo Treatments," British Medical Journal 332 (2006): 391–97.

placebo groups. Those who underwent sham acupuncture improved at a faster rate than those who received the placebo pill (Table 6). The differences are small, but the lesson is telling. A placebo pill is no match for the acupuncturist's treatment act: the rituals, the beliefs, the body language, the explanations, and whatever else went on when the needle didn't pierce the skin time after time. But a placebo pill is palliative as well. Persistent regional arm pain is as complex an illness experience as persistent regional low back pain and as worthy of the analysis we are bringing to bear on low back pain.[21] No one would sanction a placebo-controlled trial of the treatment of bacterial meningitis; knowingly treating with an ineffective regimen is criminal in that circumstance. But treating regional arm pain with a placebo in a clinical trial is laudable and instructive. It turns out the placebo is palliative, and sham acupuncture is more palliative than the placebo pill. Does that mean that sham acupuncture is no longer a placebo? The sugar pill may not be a placebo, either, since these patients improved, but the comparison is with baseline symptoms, and improvement might simply reflect passage of time. We call sham acupuncture a placebo because the procedure was designed to be a "sham" and was administered by an acupuncturist who knowingly deceived the patients; yet pain was reduced more than was observed coincident with swallowing a sugar pill.

Much is known about this placebo effect. It requires a subjective outcome that is important to the sufferer; pain perception is altered but not grip strength, which is nearly as subjective a measure (see Table 6). It requires a degree of conviction on the part of the purveyor. And it requires a degree of optimistic expectation on the part of the subject. When the expectation of the patient and the conviction of the practitioner resonate, some degree of amelioration of symptoms is the likely outcome.

Is a "good bedside manner" a placebo? It certainly has the attributes just listed. It has never been subjected to scientific testing, though perhaps it should be. After all, current reimbursement schemes do not allow for much of the time necessary to establish the trusting relationship that is prerequisite for a good bedside manner. Maybe a good bedside manner is a cost-effective approach to symptom control. If it is, would we call it a placebo effect?

The placebo effect has a negative connotation because it carries with it much "mind-body" baggage. If demeanor and conviction can conspire to palliate back pain or arm pain, the inescapable conclusion is that the pain is "in your mind." And so it is, at least in part. That does not mean there is no painful, local process at work in your low back—a local, pain-producing (nociceptive) event. However, the perception of painfulness includes an important element of cognition, particularly the suffering that overlays the pain. This cognitive component is tempered by prior experiences (or lack thereof), by preconceptions, and by anxiety. It is this plastic component of the morbidity that is amenable to palliation by "bedside manner" and by "placebo." It is this plastic component that is "in your mind." And it is this plastic component that can predominate, or be learned to predominate, if the circumstance is educational, as in tort litigation or disability determination. Such a psychological conceptualization is supported by modern neurophysiology. It is a conceptualization that is more Cartesian than the dualism typically and wrongly attributed to Descartes:

> But there is nothing which nature teaches me more expressly
> (or more sensibly) than that I have a body which is ill affected when
> I feel pain, and stands in need of food and drink when I experience
> the sensations of hunger and thirst. . . . Nature likewise teaches
> me by these sensations of pain, hunger, thirst . . . that I am not
> only lodged in my body as a pilot in a vessel, but that I am besides
> so intimately conjoined, and as it were intermixed with it, that my
> mind and body compose a certain unity. . . . [A]ll these sensations
> . . . are nothing more than certain confused modes of thinking,
> arising from the union and apparent fusion of mind and body.
> (René Descartes [1596–1650], *Meditations on First Philosophy*)

The mind-body baggage results from the contemporaneous debate on the site and substance of the soul. This is exemplified by the writings of Descartes's contemporary Blaise Pascal (1623–62), who turned his extraordinary mind away from the exquisitely analytical to mystical Jansenism and concluded the "ills of the body are nothing more than punishment for the ills of the soul."

The fact that placebo denotes "in your mind" is not troubling to me, nor should it be to anyone else anymore. I am not ashamed that I cultivate my bedside manner and that my patients feel better as a result. I neither think nor imply that anything about my demeanor is curative. I am establishing a relationship that fosters coping by my patients. I do not call this "placebo." I reserve placebo for those interventions that have any element of deception. An acupuncturist who treats a patient with regional arm pain by some meticulous ritualistic regimen of needling is purveying a placebo unless the acupuncturist can find some argument against the implications of Table 6, or the patient is made aware that it is the treatment act of the acupuncturist and not the needling that may afford some relief if he or she sees fit for it to do so. My bedside manner requires no needles or props except maybe my white coat.

Modalities and the Treatment Act

The distinction between a "treatment" and a "treatment act" is crucial to our understanding of the therapeutic alternatives that are available to people with regional low back pain in the United States and elsewhere, as well as those that were available in the past. The *treatment* is what is done to you; the *treatment act* is a therapeutic envelope in which the treatment is administered, an envelope that nearly always includes human interactions. For most of the alternatives, the treatment is generally termed a "modality," often a physical event. With rare exceptions, all modalities that have been tested (and nearly all have been tested) are no more effective than a sham alternative. Nonetheless, alternative therapies exist and persist whenever enough individuals ascribe a comforting effect of the treatment act to the modality. Those who are comforted and those who are purveyors develop a bond of conviction that escalates whenever the modality is labeled placebo, and subsequently they are accused of mind games. The patient absorbs the idioms that are peculiar to the modality and espouses the treatment act in a narrative that is both distinctive and defiant. The patient learns a new way to think about the body and its ills. He or she is changed, forever becoming an advocate of the particular form of sectarian medicine. No one with a regional musculoskeletal disorder should enter into any treatment act without forewarning, understanding, and personal choice.

Clinical Judgment and the "Art" of Medicine

Medicine is not an "art." Medicine is a philosophy; epistemology and semiotics (the meanings of such symbols as symptoms and signs) are as critical to clinical scholarship as biochemistry. However, with the flowering of the biological sciences in the twentieth century, the study of the disease came to dominate the appreciation of the person who harbored the disease. The exercise rapidly became reductionistic. The patient soon was seen to be a sum of parts and the patient's illness a result of the part that was most diseased. Reductionism had triumphs, many of which are dramatic. But these triumphs pertain to a small fraction of the burden of illness. The remainder of illness is relegated to the "someday we will understand the cause" category and treated through trial and error in an exercise termed "clinical judgment."

Clinical judgment is the wisdom that derives from the accumulation of anecdotal experiences. It is the "been there, done that," the treatments that did or did not help. Since each clinical experience is idiosyncratic to an important degree, clinical judgment is the result of a cumulative and integrative bedside memory that takes advantage of the clinical judgment of mentors and peers and is willing to be exposed to peer review and criticism. Clinical judgment is endangered by spare underwriting and a dearth of mentors.

Faced with progressive organ-system damage, we have no better option than clinical medicine. Faced with progressive organ damage for which there is no meaningful reductionistic, evidence-based treatment, we can reasonably cast about for alternatives in the absence of a comforting medical treatment act. However, faced with an illness that lacks important pathophysiological correlates, and for which there is no meaningfully effective evidence-based treatment, medicine has nothing to offer but clinical judgment. Much of the clinical judgment that bears on the regional musculoskeletal disorders in general and regional low back pain in particular has been subjected to scientific scrutiny in the past few decades. Little has escaped unscathed. No wonder that alternative, sectarian providers have come into being and thrived.

Poking, Prodding, Yanking, and Girding of Loins

I do not use the term "sectarian" as an insult. No other rubric satisfactorily indicates "organized movements seeking professional status for practitioners"[22] who do not satisfy the legal, educational, and other mainstream prerequisites I have attained. Nearly all alternative terms also imply disapproval by or opposition from the dominant group and are similarly inflammatory. The politically correct current compromise, "complementary and alternative medicine," sits poorly with me, since most forms of sectarian medicine have not been shown to be complementary nor is there any compelling reason to integrate alternative therapeutic schemes into some form of "integrative medicine." Given that my guild dominates, I am comfortable with "sectarian medicine" to describe the alternatives until such time as these sectarian practices withstand scientific testing as to their effectiveness, let alone complementarity. I admit to chauvinism; I value my profession above all others to the extent that it tests the limits of certainty regarding the validity of its therapeutic offerings. I write extensively on how the institution of contemporary medicine has lost its way, but I also write extensively on how its practitioners hear a higher calling. I use the term "guild" intentionally and advisedly, although others bridle at my willingness to cast medicine, and the alternatives, in a medieval frame of reference,[23] particularly since the medieval craft guilds' demise can be attributed to their self-serving monopolistic intransigence in the face of a developing open market.

There have always been healers willing to trample your aching back, to poke it, yank it, hug it, and all else, in all societies—and there still are. Medical luminaries of their day employed and wrote about massage, traction, and manipulation—Avicenna in the eleventh century, Charef-Ed-Din in the fifteenth century, and Ambroise Paré in the sixteenth century to name but a few. Two made-in-America examples of sectarian medicine are worthy of our attention because they thrive today and because they consider regional low back pain their purview: osteopathy and the chiropractic.

Andrew Taylor Still (1828–1917) had learned medicine by apprenticeship. He was practicing in rural Kansas when tragedy struck: his three children succumbed to meningitis in the epidemic of 1864 despite heroic measures taken by their attending physicians. Disillusioned, he set out to devise an alternative system of healing. As the son of a Methodist minister, Still believed that imbibing alcohol was sinful. If alcohol is sinful, then aren't other drugs as well? He was drawn to the theories of Anton Mesmer and the magnetic healers with their belief that diseases were caused by interruptions in the pathways for magnetic fluids in the body. The magnetic healers employed magnets to redirect that flow. Still postulated that manipulative techniques, which had long been practiced by bonesetters and the like, should work as well as magnets, if not better.

Bonesetters—nonphysicians skilled at setting fractures—were the precursors of modern orthopedists, just as barbers were the precursors of modern surgeons. Bonesetters were not above manipulating in the absence of an overt fracture, a practice that the legendary British surgeon Sir James Paget in 1867 begrudgingly acknowledged "sometimes does good."[24] Still's notion was that the manipulation would promote local blood flow and thereby healing. He founded his school of osteopathy in Kirksville, Missouri, in 1892, teaching others how to "realign displacements," or rearrange obstructing musculoskeletal segments, usually in the spine. Once the segments were realigned, natural healing could proceed without recourse to allopathic drugs. By the turn of the twentieth century, Still had an infirmary in Kirksville, over 700 graduates, and a sizable following. Osteopathic schools opened elsewhere. Patients who were under the care of osteopaths fared better than those treated to "heroic medicine" in the influenza epidemic of 1918–19. Over the objections of Still, then eighty-seven years old, the American Osteopathic Association decided to incorporate the "materia medica" of mainstream medicine into the curriculum in the early twentieth century. By the middle of the twentieth century, there were fifteen schools of osteopathic medicine with curricula similar to that of the traditional medical schools. In the early 1960s, the California Medical Association and the California Osteopathic Association merged; the College of Osteopathic Physicians and Surgeons became the University of California College of Medicine, Irvine. By the 1960s, all states licensed osteopaths with privileges comparable to those of an M.D. Nonetheless, the American Osteopathic Association maintains control over accreditation of the osteopathic schools, grants a D.O. degree, and mandates courses in musculoskeletal manipulation. Although the vitalistic theories that seduced Still are long gone, osteopathy still teaches that manipulation reduces "somatic dysfunction." Michigan State University houses curricula leading to either the M.D. or D.O. degree in the same facility, with many courses in common. Graduates of osteopathic schools often seek postgraduate training in facilities dominated by graduates of medical schools and adopt similar practice styles, relying little on manipulation if at all. The current editor of *Spine*, the preeminent journal in the field of spinal disorders, is James Weinstein, D.O., professor and chair of orthopedics at Dartmouth.

This evolution has caused some to wonder why osteopathic medicine has not been fully absorbed into orthodox medicine.[25] I had the temerity to ask that question of a number of deans of osteopathic colleges at a dinner after I had delivered a keynote address at an annual meeting of the American Osteopathic Association a decade ago. The answer was that their schools and graduates could not compete with neighboring premier medical schools without the distinctiveness of the D.O. designation.

The chiropractic and mainstream medicine have no such cozy relationship. The chiropractic was founded by a grocer in 1895 in Davenport, Iowa. Daniel David (D. D.) Palmer (1845–1913) was as messianic as Still and also into vitalism. He reasoned that excessive "tone" produced "impingement, a pressure on nerves," from which disease resulted. "Adjusting vertebrae, using the spinous and transverse processes as [a] lever," could relieve that "tone." Palmer claimed to have cured a janitor, Harvey Lilliard, of deafness by manipulating his spine on September 18, 1895. He claimed to improve heart failure by manipulation of the neck. By the turn of the twentieth century, D. D. Palmer had a school, an infirmary, students, and a moniker for his sectarian therapy: "chiropractic," which is derived from the Greek *cheir* (hand) and *praxis* (specific use). Palmer's son, B. J. Palmer, was one of his first students. B. J. later purchased the school and managed to turn it into a successful enterprise. He and his followers were proponents of pure, "straight," unadulterated chiropractic. His stridency soon begot sectarian subdivisions. "Mixers" were willing to incorporate the practices of other sects into their own—"naropaths," who treated irritated ligaments instead of impinged nerves; "neuropaths," who felt that the impingements were outside the spine; and others, such as "naturopaths" and "physiotherapists." Several of these splinter sects have faded away, but not all have, and several are making a comeback.

To this day, a schism persists in the chiropractic between "mixers" and "straights," particularly the "straight-straights" that adhere to D. D. Palmer's vitalistic theory. For example, Sid Williams, D.C., founded Life Chiropractic College and with his wife, Nell, grew it into Life University. The school occupied a large campus in the suburbs of Atlanta and achieved influence that extended as far as underwriting a committee of the World Health Organization to examine options for treating low back pain in the developing world. Sid Williams was a "straight-straight" and demagogue who was a lightning rod in the chiropractic, even to the extent that the credentialing of his university was threatened. There is an organization, the World Chiropractic Alliance, that serves as a voice for straights in contradistinction to the more inclusive American Chiropractic Association. The stated position of the World Chiropractic Alliance says it all: "The correction of subluxation is applicable to any patient exhibiting evidence of its existence regardless of the presence or absence of symptoms and disease. Therefore, the determination of the presence of subluxation may stand as the sole rationale for care." Regardless of their theoretical orientation, all chiropractors employ spinal manipulation as the primary modality and the essence of their practice.[26] Finding "subluxations," the chiropractic diagnosis that implies spinal misalignment, requires the finger of faith. Interobserver reliability in the detection of subluxations approaches nil; in other words, if two chiropractors agree on the details of the examination in this regard, it is by sheer luck. Contentious within the chiropractic, and very contentious for mainstream medicine, is the purview of the chiropractic. Is the chiropractors' purview solely the regional musculoskeletal disorders? That is not the stance of many chiropractors and many schools of chiropractic. Some chiropractors "reduce subluxations" for a range of ailments, including headache, menstrual cramps, inattentiveness, and asthma.

The bickering within the chiropractic pales next to the open warfare with the medical establishment that played out through much of the twentieth century. By midcentury the American Medical Association held the chiropractic to be quackery and declared interactions with chiropractors on a professional level to be unethical. Chiropractors thrived nonetheless and now number over 60,000 worldwide; they practice mainly in the United States, where they are third in number behind those with M.D. and D.D.S. degrees. Furthermore, chiropractors took my guild to task in the courts, so that by 1975 the chiropractic was licensed in all states; four years later, the formalized prejudice of the AMA was found to be illegal. Chiropractic treatments are indemnified by workers' compensation and Medicare.

The latest triumph of the chiropractic advocacy groups involved the Veterans Health Administration (VHA). A decade ago, Congress passed a bill that instructed the VHA to undertake a scientific study to support their policy that disallowed chiropractic practice in VHA hospitals. I was asked to review the protocol that was developed. I pointed out that the protocol was so severely flawed as to be ridiculous. Veterans suffering chronic disabling back pain were randomized to usual care in the hospital or care in a local private chiropractic office. Outcomes to be measured were satisfaction with care and decrease in disability. Both were predictable; outside care would be regarded as much more pleasant, and no veteran could be expected to agree to something that would result in a decrease in his or her disability award. To their credit, the chiropractic leadership agreed with me and my solution, which was to do the randomization in the hospital. The response of the VHA was that such was not possible since chiropractors could not practice in VHA hospitals, a catch-22. The study was done as designed, and in 2002 President Bush signed a law permitting the chiropractic access to VHA hospitals.

"Straights" and "mixers" are licensed to perform manipulative therapies and imaging studies but not to prescribe pharmaceuticals. Subluxations are imaginary; there are no such specific skeletal changes that correlate with symptoms. However, chiropractors are skilled at applying brief, high velocity force to the vertebral column sufficient to create a vacuum phenomenon in the small joints of the spinal column. The joints snap back with cracking sounds and sensations that cause chiropractors to feel accomplished and their patients to feel treated. That anyone can imagine such an event can salve asthma, or diabetes, or the like is a testimony to the tenacity of vitalistic theories in the face of a telling science.[27] When it comes to regional back pain, however, the chiropractic has staked out its turf. Two of the stakes are driven quite deeply: first, spinal manipulation as a modality may not always be a placebo; and second, many who avail themselves of the chiropractic perceive themselves better off for the efforts.

The Effectiveness of Spinal Manipulation as a Modality

I have long been fascinated by the staying power of folk remedies such as back cracking. Clearly some, and perhaps nearly all, folk remedies are simply delusional idiosyncrasies of culture. But back cracking is sufficiently distinctive to foster entire schools of sectarian medicine. Are the practitioners self-deluding and their patients seduced by placebo events? In 1973 I was the British-American Fellow of the American Heart Association and the British Heart Foundation privileged to pursue very basic research in a premier laboratory in London. I could not resist taking a weekend course in "orthopaedic medicine" in a neighboring hospital. "Orthopaedic medicine" was founded by James Cyriax, an orthopedic surgeon in London who practiced manipulative medicine similar to that promulgated by osteopathy but without vitalistic underpinnings. Cyriax's textbook went through many editions and his approach had many disciples, including at the University of Rochester in New York. To my eye, it was hocus-pocus. Peter Curtis, now retired, was a British-trained family physician who had learned

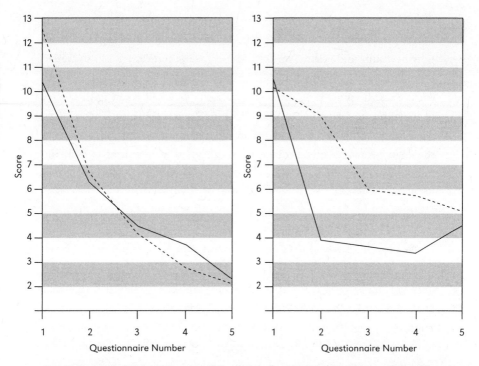

FIGURE 4. Results of the University of North Carolina Trial of Spinal Manipulation. The volunteers with regional low back pain were stratified into those who were hurting for two weeks or less (left) and two to four weeks (right). The addition of the long lever-arm, high-velocity manipulation (solid line) to mobilization (broken line) made no difference to the course of the former. However, those subjected to manipulation in the latter stratum achieved a 50 percent reduction in score more rapidly (P = 0.009). (Reprinted with permission of the publisher of *Spine* from the original publication: N. M. Hadler, P. Curtis, D. B. Gillings, and S. Stinnett, "A Benefit of Spinal Manipulation as Adjunctive Therapy for Acute Low Back Pain: A Stratified Controlled Trial," *Spine* 12 [1987]: 703–6)

orthopedic medicine in London and practiced it as a professor of family medicine on the faculty of the University of North Carolina at Chapel Hill. There, we were long colleagues, jousting and jesting about his approach to low back pain. To settle our debate, we obtained funding for a randomized controlled trial from the Robert Wood Johnson Foundation and published the results over twenty years ago.[28] The principal result is presented in Figure 4. We advertised on campus to recruit people with regional back pain of less than a month's duration for a trial comparing two forms of spinal manipulation. To be selected, a volunteer must have never undergone any form of spinal manipulation in the past and must have not been involved in any claim for disability or compensability. All sixty volunteers received a thorough examination from me designed to be most reassuring in terms of prognosis. Then Peter entered the room. He performed a form of mobilization, a rocking and flexing, on all, and then by random assignation a classic osteopathic manipulation on half. This was a long lever-arm, high-velocity back crack; he pinned one shoulder to the table while rotating the pelvis in the opposite direction, resulting in a loud cracking noise. The subjects were followed for two weeks with a validated questionnaire that assessed the degree to which their back pain interfered with activities of daily living. All were well again in two weeks. For those who were hurting for two weeks or less when they volunteered, it made no difference if Peter cracked their back. However, those who were hurting for two to four weeks experienced a 50 percent reduction in score more rapidly.

This result is reproducible if the subjects are comparably free of confounders such as chronicity and issues that relate to work incapacity. There is even some benefit if these prerequisites are relaxed slightly,[29] but that benefit is harder to reproduce.[30] There is no data that repeating the crack offers anything. Nonetheless, it is this data that led the AHCPR committee to recommend a single spinal manipulation in the treatment of acute low back pain. However, at best this is much ado about very little.[31] Certainly, it is little reason to advocate a form of sectarian medicine. I have never felt comfortable performing manipulation, recommending manipulation, or letting anyone crack my back. But no other modality has even this much scientific support.

The Effectiveness of Spinal Manipulation as Part of a Treatment Act

The North Carolina Back Pain Project was established in the early 1990s under the direction of Tim Carey and with the participation of a number of my colleagues at UNC–Chapel Hill. We recruited over 200 practices to enroll their patients with acute low back pain into a telephone survey that we continued for over a decade. Urban and rural primary care, orthopedic, and chiropractic practices were well represented by the more than 1,500 patients enrolled. The outcomes were similar at six months, but healthcare utilization was very different. Patients of chiropractors returned repeatedly to the same practitioner, a frequency that ran cost up to that of the patients of the orthopedic surgeons.[32] Whether the treatment is in a rural or urban setting, and whether it is indemnified by workers' compensation or not, those people who choose to seek the ministrations of chiropractors for low back pain tend to do so repeatedly and are more satisfied than those who choose medical practitioners. And, as I had argued before the VHA years ago, patient satisfaction is measurably palliative in the short and long term, though not dramatically so.[33] However, is this small benefit a result of something more than the "bedside manner" of a chiropractor who makes a living treating patients with low back pain as opposed to the "bedside manner" of physicians who are far less comfortable with this particular illness? If that's all there is to it, as observational data suggests,[34] teaching physicians to communicate effectively with acute-low-back-pain patients could supplant any need for patients to seek out chiropractic care.

There have been a number of trials in which the outcomes for patients with low back pain who are offered ancillary physical treatments are compared with those for patients who are not offered such ancillary treatment. If there are benefits, they are modest[35] and transient.[36] So we are left with the "bedside manner" as the explanation for why patients of chiropractors return repeatedly. Fortunately, we have important insights about this interaction. The patients of the chiropractic are predominately middle-aged, white, married people whose personal philosophic orientations and preconceptions are particularly compatible with those espoused by the chiropractic.[37] They have significantly poorer mental health than medical back pain patients.[38] Furthermore, these psychosocial attributes bode poorly in terms of persistence of pain and incidence of recurrent episodes.[39] The chiropractic may be providing a port in their storm, but one that the chiropractic seems little cognizant of nor much of a match for.

Regional Low Back Pain and the Surrogate Complaint

Manipulative sectarian medicine is not the only alternative to which patients with regional low back pain are turning. There are alternatives to this alternative that are notable for their purveyance of various physical modalities, potions, and unctions with even less in the way of scientific support. And then there are the many—more than 2 percent of all office visitors—who turn to medical doctors,[40] most of whom will report continual pain or recurrences five years later.[41]

Could it be that all this putative healing and helping is missing the forest for the trees? Could it be that many of those who seek care for their back pain are actually seeking compassionate concern for why they need to seek care? Could it be that "back pain" is a contemporary surrogate for the plaint of being overwhelmed by life's challenges when experiencing back pain? These are the themes of this book.

SIX

Invasion of the Spine Surgeons

The practice of what we call "surgery" has a long and colorful history. It has always been the remedy for wounds and tumors (classically, any swelling was a tumor, even if it was a boil or other infection). Furthermore, competence in surgeons was demanded as far back as ancient Babylon, and incompetence was severely punished: "If a physician make a large incision with an operating knife and cure it, or if he open a tumor (over the eye) with an operating knife, and saves the eye, he shall receive ten shekels in money. . . . If a physician make a large incision with the operating knife and kill him, or open a tumor with the operating knife, and cut out the eye, his hands shall be cut off" (Code of Hammurabi, circa 1760 BCE).

Perhaps it was fear of punishment that stayed the hand of prior generations of surgeons when it came to the spine.[1] Very little trepidation remains in the twenty-first century, however, particularly in the United States. The following case is illustrative. This patient's saga commences in his childhood, which was colored by multiple illnesses so that his family considered him sickly. His teenage years were notable for an inability to gain weight, easy fatiguing, periodic abdominal pain, and episodes of diarrhea. He was extensively and repeatedly evaluated by prominent physicians at Harvard, Yale, and the Mayo Clinic with no certain diagnosis but sufficient suspicion to commence corticosteroid therapy for colitis. At age twenty-three, the patient had the first of many episodes of severe low back pain. Despite recurrences of abdominal pain, diarrhea, and backache, he was an athlete through college and later gained distinction as a military officer. But because of intermittent, intense low back pain, he underwent a discectomy (removal of discal tissue), a procedure that proved to no avail. Low back pain continued to plague him, progressing in severity so that his gait was impaired. When he was thirty-seven, surgeons at Cornell attempted to fuse the lumbar spine by attaching a metal plate with screws. The postoperative course was complicated by recurrent infections, some life threatening, so that four months later the hardware was removed and replaced with bone grafts. From age thirty-seven to forty, the patient functioned despite chronic low back pain, multiple hospitalizations, frequent "trigger-point injections," bracing, and multiple pharmaceuticals. He functioned so well that in 1960 he was elected president of the United States. John F. Kennedy's tenure in the White House has been called "a thousand days of suffering" despite the ministrations of a number of in-house clinicians. JFK's medical history was assiduously hidden from public view by his family and advisers for fear that it would compromise his career as a politician. It has only recently come to light.[2]

For our purposes in this chapter, it is noteworthy that some of the leading spine surgeons in the country had the temerity to operate on JFK's spine based on their conviction that some structure had to be altered for him to experience relief. Such hubris has been called "eminence-based medicine." Clearly it was tolerated if not applauded by the peers of these surgeons at some of the nation's most prestigious medical centers. Clearly "surgical cure" seduced one of the nation's canniest of families. And clearly the eminence of the surgeons overshadowed any sense of culpability for the complications that were recognized and others that were less obvious. No one was suggesting that their hands be cut off.

Treating Low Back Pain on a Procrustean Bed

One translation of Hippocrates' *Epidemics*, book 1, section 11, reads: "As to diseases, make a habit of two things—to help, or at least to do no harm." The Greek aphorism became "first, do no harm," translated as *Primum non nocere* in Latin, which has been attributed to the Roman physician Galen. The ethic is meant to suppress the urge to prescribe treatments that had even a remote possibility of causing more harm than good. Though handed down from generation to generation of physicians ever since, this ethic has never rested easily in the medical profession. The reflex is to do something, and the more dramatic that something is, particularly if it is dangerous or painful, the more it is accepted by peers and held in awe by the laity.

My generation has stood witness to this dialectic. In the mid-twentieth century, "conservative" was still the adjective applied to therapies that were cautious yet reasonable; aggressiveness was condemned even if a rationale was articulated. By the end of the century, "conservative" was criticized and "aggressive" was applauded. When it came to surgery, the dichotomy was magnified. By the 1970s, improvements in anesthesia, postoperative care, and surgical technique had made possible almost any elective surgery, even for the frail or very ill patient. Surgery was freed up to focus on the development of new procedures with less concern about the old adage that the procedure might succeed though the patient died.

Furthermore, the public hungered for surgical miracles. The image of the surgeon as hero, capable of death-defying, innovative feats in the setting of traumatic wounds, intraoperative catastrophes, and the like, was as thrilling to the public imagination as it was seductive for surgeons. Furthermore, there is a long history of inventiveness regarding the tools of the trade: many a surgeon has had a forceps or retractor named after him or her, which are often then patented and marketed. There is also a long history of inventiveness regarding surgical procedures. However, the pace of surgical innovation escalated; new ideas that seemed reasonable to their inventor were practiced on animals and then tried on patients. There is no such thing as an "off-label" surgical technique; the surgeon at the operating table is subject only to constraints imposed by peers. The peers applauded the more aggressive and innovative among them and society rewarded them handsomely.

The laissez-faire attitude toward surgical instruments and techniques was applied to devices that could be left on or in the patient. The notion is that a device differs from a pharmaceutical because no chemical is dissolving. This notion came under scrutiny in the early 1970s, when there was a spate of failed cardiac pacemakers and complications from the Dalkon Shield intrauterine contraceptive. After several years of congressional debate and discussion, President Gerald R. Ford signed the Medical Device Amendments to the 1938 Food, Drug, and Cosmetic Act into law in 1976.[3] The amendments define devices similarly to drugs, except that devices could be classified according to their hazardous nature so that the amount of oversight could be appropriately graduated. Class I devices required no new oversight; tongue depressors, bandages, and the like had to meet manufacturing standards—"Good Manufacturing Practice" (GMP) regulations—but little else. Class II devices were wheelchairs, impact-resistant lenses, and the like that had to meet performance standards in addition to GMP. Class III devices were those that involved invading the body and had obvious potential for harm. Class III devices required premarket approval.

The standard for approval that pertained to pharmaceuticals did not seem appropriate for devices and other "things," however. In addition to the distinction drawn with pharmaceuticals in terms of their biochemistry, it was argued that the safety of devices depends largely on their being used properly. The risk/benefit ratio of an implant or anesthesia machine or glucose monitor is as much a function of its materials and engineering as its proper usage. Therefore, the FDA is willing to accept observational studies rather than the deductive gold standard for pharmaceuticals, the randomized controlled trial. Furthermore, the FDA felt some obligation to educate practitioners and patients about the safe use of devices and to exercise authority to notify and ban usage in the case of deception or risk of injury. This line of reasoning lowers the threshold for licensing devices well below that of pharmaceuticals.

The definition of a "device" is rather loose. Not all devices are inorganic gizmos such as the hardware used to fuse spines. For example, hyaluran solution was licensed as a device for use in facilitating the insertion of the artificial lens following cataract extraction, but it was licensed as a pharmaceutical to be injected into osteoarthritic knees. Only the latter licensure was based on an RCT; the former was based on observational data and surgical testimony. Hyaluran is a high-molecular-weight sugar molecule that is a constituent of joint fluid, the vitreous humor behind the ocular lens, and the cockscomb. (As an aside, hyaluran is far more important as a device used by ophthalmologists than as a drug used by rheumatologists; I don't find the RCTs the slightest bit compelling and never inject these preparations into knees.)

There is another aspect of the 1976 amendments that moves devices onto a different regulatory island. The statute essentially preempts any attempt to regulate devices by the states. This bit of legal fine print is not trivial. For example, heart patient Charles Riegel lost a suit against Medtronic in a New York court because of this fine print. He underwent a balloon angioplasty in 1996 during which the balloon ruptured, leading to a cardiac arrest, advanced cardiac support, and a coronary-artery bypass graft. The patient and his family sued Medtronic, the manufacturer of the angioplasty balloon device. The suit was denied in New York.

Poor Mr. Riegel has since died. Nonetheless, the family appealed this decision. In December 2007 the U.S. Supreme Court heard arguments in *Riegel v. Medtronic*. Whether plaintiffs who claim injury from a defective medical device are barred from a tort in state court was only one of the issues. This suit was revisiting a 1996 Supreme Court decision that FDA licensure and appropriate warnings in labeling did not preclude damages in a medical device tort.[4] In February 2008 the Supreme Court found 8 to 1 in favor of the manufacturer in *Riegel v. Medtronic*. In effect, device manufacturers have gained tort immunity based on FDA licensure, and the burden on the agency and its resources has escalated severely. In January 2009 a district court in Minnesota expanded the notion that the federal decision preempted state law. The Minnesota suit involved Medtronic again. Is Medtronic liable when the wires (leads) from the Fidelis intracardiac defibrillator break? The Minnesota court found that since the FDA licensed the defibrillator, it was to be assumed that it was licensing its components. Therefore, the FDA approval provides immunity against product-liability suits. I am not alone in my concern regarding whether the FDA would be able to assure patient safety as a unique remedy.[5] The track record in the absence of tort immunity is disconcerting enough. The track record regarding devices for the treatment of regional low back pain is an object lesson. We will return to that lesson in chapter 9.

Regional low back pain is painful—about that there is no doubt. One can fully understand the seductive nature of the inference that there is something amiss in the structure of the low back, particularly since moving the painful low back exacerbates the pain. Because there are so many changes in the structure of the spine as we age, theories abound as to what is actually hurting—what is the specific "pain generator," in the current jargon. Almost every anatomical structure in and around the spine has had its advocates for the label "pain generator." Almost every putative pain generator has evoked a locally invasive remedy, most of which are passing fancies and some of which are violent. Rather than attempt a compendium of putative pain generators, I will focus on the pain generator that has dominated thinking for seventy years: the intervertebral disc. And rather than provide a compendium of surgical inventiveness for salving the putative discal pain generator, I will provide examples of what has been done to the disc by puncturing the skin, by surgically extirpating the disc, by preventing the motion that exacerbates the pain, and by replacing the disc. This is not a treatise on surgical technique. I seek to explore the intellectual process that drives surgical inventiveness along with the social and regulatory climate that supports this surgical enterprise. We will rely on the resulting insights to inform policy considerations in later chapters.

A brief anatomy lesson is prerequisite to understanding the discal theory of regional low back pain. Figures 2 and 3 in chapter 4 provided an overview of normal spinal anatomy. Figure 5 reiterates this from a different perspective, with emphasis on the structure of the disc. Based on the considerations in Figure 6, one can see how surgical inventiveness coalesced on the poor disc.

Injecting the Disc

There have been attempts to destroy the nucleus pulposus by injection. The theory is that by so doing, the extruding, dissecting, impinging material from the nucleus will recede along with the pain it is engendering. The early attempt took advantage of some interesting science regarding enzymes. Chymopapain is an enzyme extracted from *Carica papaya*. It will digest many proteins but not collagen. Theory held that if injected into the nucleus pulposus, it would liquify the gel without damaging the annulus, an outcome termed "chemonucleolysis."

The theory was put into practice in the early 1960s by surgeons and radiologists using enzyme preparations from various suppliers. The modern FDA came into being with the Kefauver-Harris Amendments to the Food, Drug, and Cosmetics Act, which demanded proof of efficacy for licensure. Before the FDA was even ready to consider whether chemonucleolysis was a drug, however, tens of thousands of people with low back pain had undergone the procedure. In 1976 the neurosurgical service at Walter Reed Army Medical Center undertook an RCT, randomizing sixty-six men with regional low back pain to either chemonucleolysis or an intradiscal saline injection. There was no difference in outcome at two months; about half the men were better regardless of the stuff injected into their discs.[6] The FDA took note, but its attempt to halt the performance of chemonucleolysis was met with such a hue and cry by those with a vested interest in performing chemonucleolysis and patients who were convinced they had been cured that the FDA caved, licensing the Abbott Laboratories preparation of chymopapain in 1982.[7] However, the general experience with chemonucleolysis over the next decade was dismal. Whatever benefit one was willing to ascribe to the procedure in the short term was not long lived. Abbott stopped selling the licensed Chymodiactin brand of chymopapain simply because the market had ceased to exist.

Rather than dissolve the nucleus pulposus, why not cook it? Proteins, including collagen, denature when heated, thereby giving up their fine structure and shrinking into a lump or a gel. If the protruding or dissecting

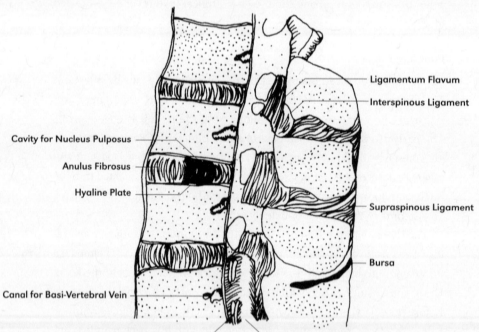

Cavity for Nucleus Pulposus

Anulus Fibrosus

Hyaline Plate

Canal for Basi-Vertebral Vein

Ligamentum Flavum

Interspinous Ligament

Supraspinous Ligament

Bursa

Ventral and Dorsal Nerve Roots

Dura Mater

FIGURE 5. This diagram views the spine as if it were cut through the center from top to bottom. The vertebral bodies are separated by the disc. The disc is a doughnut-shaped structure. The doughnut is composed of the very tough collagenous layers of the annulus fibrosus. The hole is not empty; it contains a gelatinous material, the nucleus pulposus, which is composed of a network of protein enmeshed with a network of large-strand sugar molecules. The youthful disc is a rather resilient structure that buffets compressive forces thanks to the gelatinous properties of the nucleus pulposus. The disc places constraints on the rotatory excursions of the spine by virtue of the tensile strength of the annulus. In terms of limiting the excursions of the spine, the annulus is joined by the other ligamentous structures denoted in the drawing.

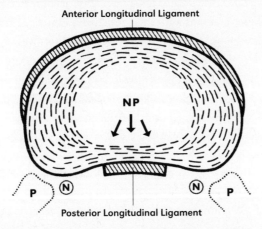

Anterior Longitudinal Ligament

NP

Posterior Longitudinal Ligament

FIGURE 6. This diagram depicts a cross section through the disc. The fibrous annulus is denoted by the hatchings. "Anterior" denotes the part of the spine pointing toward the abdominal wall and "posterior" that which is closest to the skin of the back. As we age, there is a tendency for the fibers of the annulus to disrupt so that the gelatinous nucleus pulposus (NP) dissects outwardly. It is rare for this dissection to have an anterior vector. Occasionally the vector is directly posterior toward the posterior longitudinal ligament, which bulges into the spinal canal, even impinging on the spinal cord (see Figure 5 for an appreciation of this arrangement). However, it is far more likely that the dissection of NP will have a posterolateral vector, causing the annulus to bulge, even impinging on the nerves (N) that are exiting the cord at that level. The commonest spinal level for such a posterolateral herniation of the NP is between the fifth lumbar and first sacral vertebrae, where the exiting nerve is a major part of the sciatic nerve. If that nerve is irritated or damaged, the pain radiates down the leg and the illness is termed "sciatica."

disc is the culprit, this should do the trick. Several intrepid arthroscopists played with this idea for various conditions in peripheral joints in the early 1990s with lasers and the like. It waited for the Saal brothers to invent a way to do thermal violence to the disc. Jeffrey and Joel Saal are the SOAR Physiatry Medical Group in Menlo Park, California. They invented a catheter that they could thread through a needle inserted into the center of a disc. The catheter end was a thermal-resistive coil so they could heat the nucleus to a painful 90° C. They termed the procedure "intradiscal electrothermal annuloplasty and nucleotomy," for which they coined the acronym IDET. They reported results in professional meetings, and in early 2000 they published a "preliminary report" on their first twenty-five patients.[8] Later in 2000, they published their results one year following IDET; only twelve of their carefully selected sixty-two patients with persistent low back pain were no better.[9] Saal and Saal further reported that the beneficial response was durable a year later.[10] Several others were publishing similar if not more encouraging results with IDET in patients who had not responded to anything else, even patients who were enmeshed in workers' compensation indemnification battles. For example, a report from a small practice in Eugene, Oregon, compared patients with chronic back pain who underwent IDET because their insurance company was willing to pay for it with those who were denied coverage, claiming impressive improvement in the former group.[11] Because of these and other studies, the FDA licensed the SpineCath Intradiscal Catheters, manufactured by Oratec, and even approved a modification in 1992, long before the papers were published.

All of these studies were published in *Spine*, a highly respected and oft-cited journal that was founded over thirty years ago. I have long been a member of the editorial board and am proud of that affiliation. *Spine* and all other prominent journals have tried to come to grips with the declaration of a conflict of interest by authors regarding the rationale for their studies, particularly studies of devices and pharmaceuticals. There is a footnote to each of the IDET papers that offers an assertion that the authors have received some financial benefit related to the report. The format for this admission varied over time, but in 2002 it included "benefits in some form have been or will be received from a commercial party related directly or indirectly to the subject of the manuscript."

I had no idea of the extent of the commercial involvement at the time. There was not even mention of the manufacturer of the IDET apparatus in any of these manuscripts. It turns out that Jeffrey Saal cofounded Oratec Interventions, Inc., in 1995 and served as director. By 2000 Oratec was a publicly traded company. By 2001 Oratec's annual gross income from IDET products was $21 million. Oratec counted 3,000 physicians as customers who had performed over 400,000 IDET procedures. On February 14, 2002, Smith & Nephew, a large British corporation, acquired Oratec for $310 million. All this was going on before the data describing the clinical experience was published. Furthermore, all this data is observational, and much of it is generated on the patients of physicians who stood to lose so much if the results were disappointing. If this was a pharmaceutical, it would never have been licensed on the basis of such information.

There have since been three RCTs on IDET. The best designed is a double-blind trial from Adelaide published in 2005.[12] The catheter was inserted into the disc of all subjects but the current turned on only in some, unbeknownst to the patient, the surgeon, or the evaluators. There was no difference in outcome between the sham and the actively treated patients; neither group did particularly well. But I am not sure the belated science has had much to do with the fading of the enthusiasm for IDET. It is still a licensed device, as is chymopapain. And it still has advocates, convinced they are helping their patients and touting observational data.[13] But most of the spine surgeons and interventionists have moved on to greener pastures.

Removing the Disc

While we are on the theme of very lucrative ideas that are marketed as safer and gentler than the knife for persistent low back pain, automated percutaneous lumbar discectomy (APLD) deserves mention. There have been attempts to dig out the disc with small instruments inserted through punctures in the skin since the 1970s. None seemed effective until Gary Onik invented his "Nucleotome." Onik is to APLDs what Jeffrey Saal is to IDETs. He published studies of the Nucleotome's action on cadaver spines in 1985, and in 1987 he published a paper claiming that APLD was a boon for thirty-one of thirty-six patients. He announced that APLDs were likely to replace laminectomies.[14] He also collected a group of fellow travelers, many of whom were on the masthead of the 1987 paper and from radiology departments that had started to ply this trade, with Pittsburgh as the epicenter.

By 1991 Onik could boast that more than 3,000 physicians had been trained to perform APLD and over 40,000 patients had submitted. Observational data had already been published in nineteen papers on nearly 4,000 patients, with a "success rate" consistently over 70 percent.[15] The Nucleotome passed muster with the FDA as a device. It is an electrical drill-like tool with a specialized bit that can cut and trap discal material. Clarus Medical, Inc., was founded in 2000 and manufactured and sold over 200,000 Nucleotomes in short order.

Since then, the enthusiasm for APLD has waned. There are complications, and there are far more treatment failures than would be expected from the results of the observational trials undertaken in the zeal for the novelty of APLD. There has been no elegant trial as there was for IDET, a sham-controlled trial, but there have been a number of RCTs. My favorite was orchestrated by my friend and colleague Michel Revel of Hôpital Cochin in Paris. In this multicenter trial, APLD was not associated even with as much short-term benefit as chemonucleolysis,[16] and we have already considered the "benefit" to be derived from chemonucleolysis. Furthermore, in this trial, about a third of the patients improved regardless of the intervention. That is nowhere near the 70 percent "success rate" claimed by those doing the observational trials that foisted APLD on the public.

How many more waves of therapeutic zeal must we witness—waves of spine-surgical inventiveness that provide nothing more than testimony to hubris and often greed—before we design a way to abort the next? I am even more strident about interventional cardiology,[17] but spine surgery is second on my list of medical specialties that are ethically challenged. I will consider structural remedies for this sad state of affairs in the last chapter. For now, I'll bemoan the erosion of professionalism and the corrosion of the moral compass of the profession I chose and which I revere for its potential good.

Laminectomy is an ancient procedure. Leon Wiltse,[18] in his elegant discourse on the history of spinal disorders, argues that Paul of Aegina was the first to describe the procedure in the seventh century CE. Many surgeons recorded doing laminectomies in the centuries that followed, usually to treat wounds or remove foreign bodies, but seldom successfully until the advent of antibiotics. The reason laminectomy dominates the field of spinal surgery is obvious if one considers spinal anatomy. Glance back at Figure 3.

Lamina is the bony plate that bears the spinous process and that forms the roof of the spinal canal. There is nothing between the skin of the back and the lamina but the paraspinous muscles, which can be retracted allowing the surgeon access to the lamina. Furthermore, removing the lamina provides access to the spinal canal without dramatically destabilizing the spine; the remaining muscles, ligaments, and facet joints are a match for that task. Once the lamina is removed, the surgeon comes upon the dural sac, which contains the spinal fluid, the spinal cord, and the nerves as they peel off from the cord at every spinal level. The spinal cord itself stops at the base of the chest. In the lumbar spine, the dural sac contains only nerve roots destined for structures in the pelvis and lower extremities. These nerves are floating in the sac like a horse's tail; hence, they are called the "cauda equina." The surgeon only has to push the dural sac aside (gently so as not to stretch the roots as they exit) to gain access to the floor of the spinal canal, which is made up of the discs and vertebral bodies encased in various ligaments. Laminectomy is the easiest and safest way to get to these structures. All other surgical approaches, and many insertions of needles and catheters, must contend with lots of vital structures that are contiguous to all other aspects of the spine, including large blood vessels, entanglements of nerves, and the bowel if one chooses to approach from the abdomen.

The disc has been well-known to anatomists for centuries. The association between discal pathology and symptoms, however, remained elusive until the pronouncements of William J. Mixter and Joseph S. Barr at the Massachusetts General Hospital in the 1930s. Mixter and Barr took advantage of laminectomy to access the disc in order to remove discal tissue (a discectomy). Thus began the "dynasty of the disc."[19] Ever since, surgeons around the developed world have studied the disc and sought ways to bring it to heel for the sake of the patient with regional low back pain or with regional sciatica. By 1940 Grafton Love at the Mayo Clinic had fine-tuned the removal of the disc by virtue of laminectomy or even "keyhole" laminotomy,[20] which was the precursor of the microdiscectomy developed by Robert Williams in Las Vegas in 1979.[21] If the disc is the evil pain generator, removing the disc should be curative. No one questioned this credo; the peer review of the treatment focused on technical matters in the operation. Questioning the credo was heresy and to a large extent is heresy still.

I have no problem questioning the credo. As we noted earlier, there is no pathology at the disc that is specific or sensitive for regional back pain. No matter what the disc looks like, a person can be asymptomatic and usually is. No one has a reliable and valid way to distinguish the disc that is hurting, despite generations of inventiveness. There is no feature of MRI that is specific enough to be diagnostic, including high-intensity zones thought by some to indicate the site of discal penetration into the annulus.[22] There is no way to render discography (injecting the disc to see if the pain can be reproduced) specific, either.[23]

All this places the discal hypothesis in a new light. The disc may be a pain generator, but we have no way to identify the particular disc that is generating the pain in a given patient. That being the case, if laminectomy/discectomy is effective in reducing the pain, it is by virtue of sheer luck. Nonetheless, spine surgeons around the world are more than willing to offer laminectomy with discectomy to their patients. Nowhere is this remedy pursued with as much vigor as in the United States, which has the highest rate of spine surgery in the world by far.[24]

The most accessible data in the United States for the rate of laminectomy/discectomy is Medicare claims data. Obviously, this data is skewed toward the elderly. Since so many of the issues we are addressing relate to working-age adults, Medicare data is less than suitable for our purposes. Unfortunately, no other data set is as accessible, reliable, or complete. The discectomy/laminectomy rate in the Medicare population has been remarkably stable for some time (we will discuss fusion surgery separately below);[25] for every 1,000 Medicare enrollees, 2.1 are discharged from the hospital following a discectomy/laminectomy each year at a cost of nearly half a billion dollars.

But that is only part of the story. It turns out that the laminectomy rate is anything but uniform across the nation. It varied eightfold in 2003, with such towns as Mason City, Iowa; Slidell, Louisiana; Casper, Wyoming; Bend, Oregon; and Billings, Montana, leading the pack and New York City and South Bend, Indiana, bringing up the rear. For years now, John Wennberg and his collaborators at the Center for the Evaluative Clinical Sciences at Dartmouth Medical School have been parsing the influences that might explain the "surgical signature" of geographic regions with some emphasis on musculoskeletal health care, spine surgery in particular.[26] The variation is not likely to reflect patient preferences given the remarkable near-neighbor geographic differences. The variation is not likely to reflect the quality of the clinical presentation, either. The better bet to explain regional differences is the density of spine surgeons and their willingness to cut (practice "styles").

A decade ago, all this violence to lamina and discs was pursued under the banner of heuristics. Discectomy was common practice. The only science that tested this belief was a quasi-controlled trial from Oslo conducted by a courageous surgeon, Henrik Weber, and published in 1983.[27] There are methodological issues with the trial in terms of allocation to the treated groups, dropouts, and crossovers. Nonetheless, there was not a hint of benefit from surgery for low back pain in the short or long term; both surgically treated and nonsurgically treated patients improved to the same degree at the same rate. (There was a hint of benefit for sciatica, or leg pain.) Little heed was paid to the implications of this trial. And little heed was paid to the stentorian voice of another pioneering Scandinavian spine surgeon, the late Alf Nachemson, who was the founding editor of the journal *Spine* and who strutted the international stage of spine surgery both as speaker and author. In 1996 Nachemson concluded that for regional low back pain, one should "never treat with surgery."[28] I had published the same conclusion repeatedly over the previous decade. But the surgical community found plenty of reasons, usually stated as different and newer surgical techniques and indications, to justify surgical hubris.

More remarkable is the fashion in which the spine surgical community can still justify their common practice even in the face of good evidence to the contrary. An RCT from Finland should have dampened their enthusiasm.[29] There were no clinically significant differences between the patients who underwent microdiscectomy and those allocated conservative management over the two-year follow-up—no difference in leg- or back-pain intensity, subjective disability, or health-related quality of life. The Dutch have published an RCT of microdiscectomy versus prolonged conservative treatment for sciatica.[30] At one year the outcomes were similar, though there was a suggestion of short-term benefit from surgery for those with leg pain. Both of these trials are exemplary by methodological criteria.

Many might wonder if the practice styles, patient expectations, and indemnification schemes in Finland and the Netherlands are so different from those in the United States that these results might not pertain. The Spine Patient Outcomes Research Trial (SPORT) is reassuring on this point.[31] This multicenter U.S. trial recruited 501 surgical candidates with persistent regional back pain and symptoms of radiculopathy (such as muscle weakness, tingling in the foot, or loss of reflexes) in a leg. The candidates were randomized to surgical discectomy or conservative therapy. Both groups improved substantially over a two-year period. Unlike the Dutch and Finnish trials, many volunteer patients in the U.S. trial allocated to conservative treatment had second thoughts (perhaps reflecting a bias in their clinical setting) and opted instead for surgery. Furthermore, another 743 candidates refused to be randomized; they were followed regardless of the treatments they elected. Because of the difficulties in recruiting volunteers into the RCT and the crossovers opted by those recruited, detailed statistical analysis is problematic. The authors argue that those undergoing surgery may have benefited in terms of their radiculopathy.[32] Nonetheless, SPORT renders quite tenuous the arguments that the Dutch and Finnish trials do not pertain to the United States. There is the suggestion that discectomy may offer a slight advantage over conservative care for radiculopathy (leg symptoms), but not for regional low back pain.[33]

Fusing the Spine

Spine surgeons, and many other surgeons, vote with their scalpels. They had only to look around the waiting room to know that discectomy was not the solution for many of their patients. No one questioned whether the disc was the pain generator. No one questioned the belief that removing the disc is palliative. Discectomy is more than an act of faith; it is a self-evident, unassailable maxim. Yet so many patients still hurt after this putative pain generator has been savaged. Something must be amiss with the procedure, not the theory. I mentioned above that laminectomy did not result in a dramatically unstable spine. Starting in the mid-twentieth century, spine surgeons began to wonder if discectomy was unsuccessful because laminectomy resulted in a degree of abnormal spine motion, which became a new pain generator. Since the early twentieth century, spine surgeons had been developing ways to fuse spines rendered unstable by traumatic injury. Hence, a theory and a technology came together to usher in the era of spinal fusion. The fusion was accomplished by harvesting bone, first from the leg and later from the iliac crest, and attaching that bone to structures above and below the laminectomy. Pioneers included Richard Rothman in Philadelphia[34] and John Frymoyer[35] in Burlington, Vermont. More and more, particularly in the United States, laminectomy/discectomy was topped off with a spinal fusion.

Of course, the early experience was felt to be very encouraging by the pioneers, so encouraging that once again a new credo was born: if fusion didn't work, it was because the fusion failed and not because fusing was a bad idea. Failure of fusion was a well-known complication in the trauma literature. Trauma surgeons were taking to fusing the more severe fractures with metal rods and screws to avert the failure that often resulted when bone grafts were used. One of the pioneers in screwing hardware into the spines of failed discectomy patients was Phillip Wilson Sr. of the Hospital for Special Surgery in New York City. In fact, it was Wilson who had the temerity to screw up Jack Kennedy's back, nearly killing him in the process.[36] A Parisian surgeon, Raymond Roy-Camille, perfected this approach by designing hardware so that metal plates could be screwed into place pedicle to pedicle, which became the standard internal fixation device for several decades.[37] Then the flood gates opened. Myriad widgets have come onto the market, various plates and cages that are introduced from all imaginable surgical approaches. Many demand extraordinary surgical skills and run terrifying surgical risks. But there are many available, and all that are available are licensed by the FDA as devices.

I mentioned above that the laminectomy/discectomy rates in the Medicare population have been relatively stable, though they are excessive when compared to other countries. The trend in lumbar fusion is rapidly escalating,[38] equaling the rate of and cost for discectomy without fusion by 2003. The literature is full of RCTs of fusion, but nearly all these trials simply compare one form of device with another, elicit all sorts of declarations of potential conflict of interest on the part of the investigators, and generally have industry support. As is true of many other medical and surgical marketplaces, it is easy to show that industry-funded studies of spine surgery devices have a significantly greater likelihood of reporting positive results than studies with any other funding source.[39] Fortunately, we have four RCTs that are not device-device trials, some of which are not tainted by overt conflicts of interest.

The breakthrough RCT of the effectiveness of fusion was published by the Swedish Lumbar Spine Study Group in 2001.[40] This was an industry-supported, multicenter RCT of several forms of fusion versus "usual nonoperative" care. Nearly 300 working-age patients with at least two years of low back pain were recruited and randomized so that 222 underwent fusion. The surgical group fared statistically and clinically better than the conservative group for the first six months, after which the difference diminished. The trial generated much discussion, particularly about the adequacy of "usual nonoperative" care as the referent group and the rather loose definition of chronic low back pain.[41] The problem with interpreting a short-term benefit from surgery relates to the dramatic nature of the surgical event rather than to the procedure itself. That is why a sham-operated control is the most powerful design. One has concerns as to whether usual care can control for the *Sturm und Drang* of a surgical event. But there is no doubt that the Swedish study elevated the debate on the effectiveness of fusion surgery and set the precedent for better trials.

J. I. Brox and several of his colleagues stepped up to the plate with a government-funded, multicenter RCT in Norway.[42] The design was similar to the Swedish trial, but the referent group underwent a specially designed program of cognitive intervention and exercises. The patients improved to the same degree and at the same rate whether they underwent fusion with posterior transpedicular screws (the type of fixation introduced by Roy-Camille) or informational sessions designed to be reassuring and to encourage activity.

The British weighed in with a government-funded, multicenter RCT comparing a specially designed intensive rehabilitation program with fusion surgery.[43] They randomized nearly 350 patients equally to undergo whatever fusion procedure the surgeon preferred or a specially designed daily outpatient program of education and exercise for three weeks. Both groups improved over the course of the next two years, but there was no important difference in the rate or degree of improvement.

Prominent investigators from various disciplines have taken pen in hand and published articles in very prominent medical journals calling for a rethinking of the use of surgery for regional low back pain, if not a moratorium on laminectomy/discectomy with or without fusion.[44] There is waffling on the question of whether surgery is effective for sciatica (leg pain), a topic that demands discussion of the degree of benefit, which we will undertake in chapter 9. However, there is little waffling on its use to treat regional low back pain, even by the Cochrane Collaboration.[45]

All this chest beating has had little effect, if any, on the rate of increase of spine surgery in the United States. The pen may be mightier than the sword, but it is not mightier than the dollar. Reed Abelson wrote a very telling essay in the *New York Times* titled "The Spine as a Profit Center."[46] She pointed out that spine-fusion surgery is one of the most lucrative areas of medicine. A single screw for attaching metal to the pedicles can cost $1,000. No wonder dozens of start-ups are joining the dozens of established companies manufacturing spine-fusion devices, most privately owned so that the participation of spine surgeons in the enterprise is not readily determinable. The kickbacks and other financial entanglements are not far from the surface, however.

In the *New York Times* article, Abelson discusses Allez Spine of Irvine, California, which has a business model that recruited spine surgeons both as investors/owners and as "its customer base." Allez and Tenet Healthcare, a hospital chain with staff surgeons who are Allez investors, defend the contractual relationships between surgeons and the companies whose products they might use in surgery by asserting that the relationships are disclosed. I find such relationships indefensible. At the request of the editor of the AMA *News*, I wrote an essay arguing that physicians should never need to disclose such relationships because if they perceive they might have such a conflict of interest, they should not care for that patient. "Disclosure should not seem necessary," I wrote, "and never is sufficient."[47]

Entrepreneurship and patient-care entanglements are not peculiar to spine surgeons. However, spine surgery is offering up an easy target for those of us for whom professionalism and ethics are irretrievably fused. Spine surgeons have been at the forefront in founding physician-owned hospitals and clinics, arguing that concentrating skills in this fashion is good for their patients. If anyone is fooled by such an argument, they need to read the analysis by Jean Mitchell.[48] Mitchell, an economist at Georgetown University, used data from workers' compensation claims to examine trends in spine treatment after the entry of physician-owned specialty clinics into Oklahoma. The founding of these enterprises was followed by a fiftyfold increase in the performance of more expensive and lucrative spinal fusions, with some decrease in the rate of the older standby procedures.

Mitchell went on to compare the rate of increase of these complex fusions in Medicare populations across the states. In New England, where physician-owned specialty hospitals are scarce, use of those procedures increased nearly 200 percent between 2000 and 2004. In states with many such physician-owned enterprises, however, the rate of increase was much higher; in Oklahoma and Arizona, for example, it was nearly 700 percent, and in Kansas the increase was nearly 1,400 percent.

Furthermore, do not assume that increased fees for service from this increase in utilization are the only source of increased revenues for these spine surgeons. Take the example of my Harvard Medical School classmate Stephen Hochschuler, one of the founding partners of the Texas Back Institute outside of Dallas, which is one of the largest spine clinics in the world. Hochschuler assumed the role of chairman of the scientific advisory board of Alphatec, a start-up in the spine surgical-widget industry. When Alphatec went public in 2007, Hochschuler received a restricted stock grant that was worth over $600,000. He is quoted by Reed Abelson in the aforementioned *New York Times* article as meriting this largesse for "involvement in the development of surgical devices."

Entrepreneurial relationships that might compromise the choice of what's best for one's patients walk a very fine line between the sanctioned and the illegal. In July 2006 Medtronic paid $40 million to settle a whistle-blower suit in federal court for allegedly paying kickbacks to induce doctors to use its spinal implants. In the fall of 2007, four manufacturers of hip and knee surgical implants (Zimmer, Inc.; DePuy Orthopaedics, Inc.; Smith & Nephew, Inc.; and Biomet Orthopedics, Inc.) faced criminal complaints in federal court for using consulting agreements with orthopedic surgeons as vehicles to induce surgeons to use their companies' products. The four companies paid a combined $311 million in fines and agreed to the appointment of federal compliance officers. And then there is the case of Patrick Chan, a forty-three-year-old Arkansas neurosurgeon who pleaded guilty on January 3, 2008, in the U.S. Eastern District of Arkansas courtroom to soliciting and receiving kickbacks from a sales representative purveying spine surgery hardware for Blackstone, a U.S. subsidiary of the Dutch company Orthofix International. This, too, was a whistle-blower suit, and the whistle-blower was the sales representative for Medtronic, a competitor of Blackstone.

Artificial Disks

As I said before, spine surgeons, and many other surgeons, vote with their scalpels. Few of them doubt that the "pain generator" is in the disc, but more and more have begun to question the effectiveness of discectomy, even with fusion. Fusion may stop the motion of the discal pain generator, but it does not stop the pain, not even the exacerbation of pain with motion of the spine. Perhaps that is because fusion causes discs above and below the fused disc to degenerate more rapidly. Maybe, they reasoned, fusion after discectomy is the wrong idea. The discal pain generator should be removed and replaced with something that reestablishes movement. Enter the artificial disc and the procedure to insert it, the disc arthroplasty. This is technically demanding surgery fraught with potential complications. Furthermore, if the arthroplasty fails, the fallback procedures are fearsome to contemplate. Yet spine surgeons are flocking to learn how to do disc arthroplasties.

Two artificial discs have been approved by the FDA.[49] The Charité artificial disc was licensed in 2004 and is marketed by DePuy Spine, Inc., a subsidiary of Johnson & Johnson. The ProDisc was licensed on August 14, 2006, and is manufactured by Synthes Spine, Inc., a German company with its U.S. office in West Chester, Pa. They are different marvels of engineering but have much in common. So far, all the available trial data derives from company-sponsored trials comparing disc arthroplasty with spinal-fusion procedures. There have been a number of such trials of the Charité disc. All of them have relatively short-term follow-up, carefully select operative candidates, and find no important differences in outcome between fusion and arthroplasty. These "trials" are also a form of marketing: surgeons are compensated by health-insurance companies to perform the procedure, they become familiar with the particular procedure in the process, and they are often further rewarded by the purveyor for their participation in the trial and their willingness to "educate" others as to their experience.

ProDisc was licensed based on a multicenter, prospective RCT that purported to show more benefit from disc arthroplasty over the course of two years than circumferential instrumented fusion. Nearly forty surgeons were involved at seventeen centers. About 250 patients with diseased discs were randomized. The published report claimed no "major complications."[50] Furthermore, on multiple measures, the vast majority of the patients who submitted to disc arthroplasty showed improvement, whereas about 10 percent fewer of the fused patients showed improvement. In triumph, the ProDisc was declared "to be superior to circumferential fusion by multiple clinical criteria." The lead author on this paper is Jack Zigler, a partner of Stephen Hochschuler at the Texas Back Institute. The disclaimer on the paper stated that no funds were received to support the study although several authors had financial interests. Zigler was clearly quite familiar with the legal issues as he had coauthored a paper on the nuances of the FDA's device-approval process with his son, Jeffrey, and another lawyer, John Walsh.[51] Jeffrey Zigler is a "regulatory consultant" with Musculoskeletal Clinical Regulatory Advisers (MCRA), which was founded in 2000 as a private consulting firm to assist device manufacturers in their applications before the FDA. Walsh is a regulatory attorney with Synthes, a client of MCRA.

My suspicion was that the ProDisc trial result was too good to be true. After all, these patients had failed "conservative" treatment for six months and were subjected to a fusion procedure that was not likely to have benefited them. Yet they did awfully well, and those on ProDisc did even better. Enter Reed Abelson again, this time with an exposé in the *New York Times* titled "Financial Ties Are Cited as Issue in Spine Study."[52] It turns out that Zigler and doctors at about half of the seventeen research sites involved in this study stood to profit financially if ProDisc succeeded. A venture-capital fund run by the Texas Back Institute and some of the Texas Back surgeons were early-stage investors in a company that was bought by Synthes. All this came out in a patient's lawsuit. Synthes would not comment on whether the FDA had been fully informed of the potential conflicts of interest of the participating surgeons as required in the application that led to approval. FDA rules allow investigators to have financial ties with the maker of the device or drug they are studying or asked to advise about, as long as such relationships are fully disclosed. The FDA is currently revisiting the disclosures in this case, as well as the reason fifty "training cases" and 10 percent of the cases not considered "training" were excluded in the data analysis presented to the FDA.

Thousands of patients worldwide have had a ProDisc placed in their backs, each purchased for about $10,000. In the United States, Medicare and some private insurers refuse to pay for disc arthroplasty. No doubt Medicare will find itself under pressure from industry and advocacy groups to indemnify this surgery. There is some push back, even from spine surgeons, particularly a splinter group that formed the Association for Ethics in Spine Surgery. I advocate reform of the device-approval process as part of an overhaul of the FDA's licensing process as detailed in chapter 9.

SEVEN

Backbreaking Work

Altruism has an uneven history. The Judeo-Christian-Islamic tradition demands the giving of charity. In the Old Testament, *tzedakah* (the Hebrew word for "charity") is a duty, an act of justice and righteousness even for those who are not wealthy. The receiving of *tzedakah* is a right, an obligation according to Maimonides, of the needy. Almsgiving is one of the Five Pillars of Islam. Nowhere in these great traditions is poverty a crime. Poverty is a misfortune; the poor are unfortunate and deserving of charity. The history of the provision of such, prior to the welfare state, was uneven to say the least.[1]

In medieval Europe, charity was noblesse oblige. With the growth of cities, the church assumed the obligation. To do so, it evolved into a more public agency that supported medieval hospitals that served the ill, weary travelers, orphans, the aged, and the destitute. After the Protestant Reformation, this responsibility fell upon civil authorities. The most famous of the statutes that resulted were the Elizabethan Poor Laws, which survived nearly three centuries with only minor modifications.[2] The gentry appointed agents who dispensed tax revenues for public assistance. Instead of a nobleman or a priest, a functionary was charged with providing sustenance for those deemed deserving, the worthy poor.

The tradition of charity probably always had such a proviso, but it was codified in statutes such as the Poor Laws: charity was not simply for the poor; it was for the worthy poor. The Henrician Poor Law of 1536 provided relief for the worthy, jobs for the unemployed, and violent punishment for beggars. The American colonies had poor laws as well. Usually they stipulated that vagrants were to be "warned away" and punished severely if they returned. The colonies were imbued with Calvinistic fervor and had little charity, particularly toward "sturdy beggars." Cotton Mather declared: "For those who indulge themselves in idleness, the express command of God unto us is that we should let them starve."

In 1824 the legislation of New York State undertook an assessment of the scope of its public-assistance programs. The Yates Report condemned these programs for underwriting "vice, dissipation, disease and crime" by throwing the able-bodied poor into workhouses and poorhouses. An 1850 legislative committee report described the treatment of the poor in these facilities: "common domestic animals are usually more humanely provided for than the paupers in some of these institutions." Almshouses, the forerunner of the municipal hospitals, served as the dumping ground for the ill and the lame along with the able-bodied poor.[3]

George Orwell observed that one out of three working men was doomed to die a ward of the state, wretchedly in a poorhouse or alone, "slow, smelly and painful . . . like animals."[4] In 1902 Jack London dressed himself in tatters and went down into the underworld of East London to experience the life of the destitute.

> The unfit and the unneeded! The miserable and despised and for-
> gotten, dying in the social shambles. The progeny of prostitution—
> of the prostitution of men and women and children, of flesh and
> blood, and sparkle and spirit; in brief the prostitution of labor.
> If this is the best that civilization can do for the human, then give
> us howling and naked savagery. Far better to be a people of the
> wilderness and desert, of the cave and the squatting-place, than
> to be a people of the machine and the Abyss.[5]

Henry Mayhew would be a long-forgotten Victorian dandy and editor of *Punch* had he not decided to undertake a survey of the street people of London who were attempting to eke out enough money by peddling to afford bread, grog, and a room in a rooming house. If they were not successful, thievery and prostitution were options, or they could petition for entry into a poorhouse. Fecundity and longevity were not issues for them. They were a sizeable population, estimated to be about 15 percent of the population of London, the largest of industrialized cities. In 1861–62 Mayhew published the four volumes of *London Labour and the London Poor*,[6] in which he categorized the street people into those who could work, those who could not, and those who would not. The first group, the unemployed, was dismissed as a societal necessity; it was held that some percentage of the workforce should be unemployed and seeking employment so that the employed would be compliant out of fear of such a fate. The second group was the disabled, a group that Mayhew had difficulty defining. For example, he did not consider a blind person disabled if he or she was successful at panhandling. The third group was the unworthy poor, deserving of their dismal fate on the streets.

The poor laws were a window on the contingent nature of Western altruism. A petition for the meager relief they provided could be denied based solely on subjective assessments of an individual's worthiness. The ultimate reproach was voiced by David Lloyd George, chancellor of the exchequer, in a speech in Birmingham, England, on June 11, 1911: "There is no greater heroism in history, as you find in the humble annals of those who fight through life against odds to maintain their self-respect and independence. They will suffer the last privation before they pin the badge of pauperism over their hearts, and certainly before they will put it on the breast of their children."[7] The industrial world entered the twentieth century seething with social unrest. A sizeable population in all industrialized cities lived out their short lives on the streets. Furthermore, nearly all others feared such a fate should their wage-earning capacity be compromised by injury, infirmity, redundancy, or the death of the family wage earner. It mattered not whether work capacity was compromised by an injury that occurred on the job and by accident. The Industrial Revolution was dangerous. Its "human cost" was decried by Woodrow Wilson in his first inaugural address on March 4, 1913. Disabling violent injuries and even death stalked the workplace. But under the common law "unholy trinity of defenses," the worker faced a nearly insurmountable disadvantage in gaining any redress from an employer or from the state. This "unholy trinity of defenses" stood in the way.[8] First, under the doctrine of contributory negligence, the injured worker could not recover if he himself had been negligent to any degree, regardless of the extent of the employer's negligence. Under the fellow-servant doctrine, the injured worker could not recover if it could be shown that the injury had resulted from the negligence of a fellow worker, including a supervisor. And the doctrine of assumption of risk meant that the injured worker could not recover if injury was due to an inherent hazard of the job of which he had, or should have had, advance knowledge.

This era saw the birth of the plaintiff's bar and the union movement and nurtured the likes of Upton Sinclair, Karl Marx, Friedrich Engels, Ferdinand Lassalle, and many more. The English "Friendly Societies" and the Prussian

"Krankenkassen" were trade-based institutions that allowed advantaged workers to purchase insurance that would provide some "sick pay," but not medical treatment, should illness force them out of work. Workers went into debt attempting to pay medical bills, and medical practice was plagued with accounts receivable. Some workers could afford insurance that would spare their families the cost of their burial, but most could not afford even this meager assurance and almost no one could afford to insure against catastrophe. The result was the fashioning of a political solution that dominates thinking to this day.

The Prussian Welfare Monarchy

More than a century ago, Europe was in the throes of social reformation. Looming large on this stage was Otto von Bismarck's response to the progressive reformists, the creation of a "welfare monarchy" in order to "demonstrate that the state had more to offer to the working class than the Social Democrats . . . and that he expected the beneficiaries of his policy to see the light and to abandon their false friends."[9] The Prussian solution to the plight of the disadvantaged proved the template for the industrializing world, including the United States. It is important to emphasize that this was an exercise in authoritarian paternalism. Public assistance was viewed as compensation for failure in citizenship rather than as an entitlement.[10]

The Reichstag passed the Sickness Insurance Act in 1883, the Accident Insurance Law in 1884, and Old Age and Disability Insurance in 1889, defraying most of the costs by levying employers. By the turn of the century, Prussia had a national health-insurance scheme and a national old-age pension scheme. It also had in place a stratified disability scheme that became the precedent for the industrialized world and remains so today. The scheme is outlined in Table 7. Moneys for medical care and rehabilitation were not an issue in this scheme since all citizens were indemnified by other national indemnity programs. At issue was the magnitude of award. Only workers' compensation offered wage replacement. The notion was that no injured worker should suffer a loss in wage earnings even though he or she suffered a loss in wage-earning capacity as a consequence of an injury that arose out of and in the course of working. If the loss in wage-earning capacity was a consequence of a disease such as rheumatoid arthritis, the worker was still worthy but not completely worthy. If the worker could not earn enough even to meet some defined adequate standard of living, then he did not have to work but would still receive a pension (called

TABLE 7. The Prussian Disability-Insurance Scheme

LEVEL OF WORTHINESS	INSURANCE FUND	INDEMNIFICATION
Work incapacity as a consequence of a work-related injury	Workmen's accident insurance	Wage replacement and permanent partial awards
Work incapacity as a consequence of illness in a wage earner	Public pension insurance (invalid pension)	Wage replacement for a finite period then a limited award only if incapable of any work
Work incapacity in one who was never a substantial wage earner	Public aid	Subsistence award

an Invalid Pension) that allowed for an adequate standard of living. If the person was so incapacitated that he or she could not maintain even this standard yet had never been much of a wage earner, the award was even less under Public Aid. This scheme remains the codification of the "worthiness test."

Legislature after legislature across Europe followed the Prussian precedent to craft programs that pension the elderly and care for the ill and disabled. In England, David Lloyd George and William John Braithwaite, a civil servant and Lloyd George's personal assistant, followed these developments closely. The British scheme was introduced for some workers in 1911 and extended to all in 1920.[11] Workers, employers, and the state each paid contributions to a fund that would be used to grant sickness and unemployment benefits designed in such a way to keep a worker in reasonable fitness; benefits were particularly generous where local authorities were faced with pressure from the Labour movement. Some governments modified the Prussian scheme in interesting ways.[12] The Dutch, for example, were not taken by the accident distinction and indemnified work incapacity similarly, regardless of the cause.[13] On the other hand, Switzerland and New Zealand were smitten by the accident notion and expanded that stratum to encompass work incapacity resulting from an accidental injury that occurred anywhere, from motor vehicle accidents to recreational sports injuries.

THE SPEENHAMLAND EXPERIMENT AND THE NOTION OF A CITIZEN'S DIVIDEND

Almost all recourse for the able-bodied and disabled poor in the West has been contingent upon some test of "worthiness," an arbitrary test at best but often laden with prejudices. However, in the colonial era, the British undertook a social experiment in an alternative to the worthiness test: a "means test." On May 6, 1795, several justices of Berkshire and other men of power met in the Pelican Inn in Speenhamland (now part of Newbury) to consider solutions to a pressing social problem. The rural poor, not just the infirm but also the able-bodied, were desperate. True, Britain was growing a powerful empire to fuel its embryonic industrial infrastructure. But Britain also had recently suffered the loss of her American colonies and embarked on yet another war with France. The economy did not favor the agricultural laborer, who was to see open access to planting fields restricted while the cost of food rose precipitously. Many came to rely on charity from the rich; the poor laws were a terrifying and often Sisyphean fallback. Hence, many were forced to pilfer to survive, and those that were caught became the "criminals" that populated British penal colonies in Sydney, Australia, and elsewhere. The justices and gentry emerged from the Pelican Inn to pass into law the "Speenhamland system," which was embraced by magistrates across the agricultural south of England until its demise in 1834 (M. Speizman, "Speenhamland: An Experiment in Guaranteed Income," *Social Service Review* 40 [1966]: 44–55). It was felt that an adequate minimum wage should be suggested to farmers, even encouraged, but should not be enforced. Rather, if a laborer's earnings were insufficient to meet minimum subsistence requirements, the difference between wages and needs would be paid out of the "poor rate," a general tax-based source of revenue. The Speenhamland system seduced so many jurisdictions because it further stipulated the level of the safety net: the necessary minimum was calculated on the basis of the current price of a "gallon-loaf" of bread and the number of such loafs deemed necessary to feed a man and his family. Thus was born the principle of a guaranteed income. Worthiness was not the issue, just income maintenance adjusted for the cost of bread. William Pitt's Parliament was soon to pass an enabling act. This also is the origins of the notion of a "poverty level," which, to this day, is defined as a multiple of the money necessary for subsistence (usually three times that amount).

The Speenhamland system existed for thirty-nine years in spite of continuous controversy and debate. It was argued that employers had no incentive to pay a living wage since the burden of falling short was distributed among all the "ratepayers," including those who employed no laborers. They may have had less than no incentive. The Gilbert Act was legislated in 1782 to ease some of the harshness of the poor laws. Prior to the Gilbert Act, any laborer seeking charity and deemed able-bodied would find he was groveling in a "workhouse." The Gilbert Act empowered parishes to find employment for such wards outside the workhouse. These "roundsmen" represented a pool of very cheap labor, sparing the employer the issue of adequately compensating a worker under the Speenhamland system. One wonders if the Yates Report mentioned above was driven by this brutally regressive, Malthusian precedent. However, the Speenhamland system, not the Gilbert Act, is forever tainted with blame for perverting the character and resourcefulness of the English working class. Furthermore, the concept of a "guaranteed income" still bears the taint of the Speenhamland experiment. There remain scholars and politicians who are quick to champion the moral fiber of the working man and decry the ethic of employers who were willing to take advantage of the flaws that beleaguered the Speenhamland system. What is clear is that there were too many confounders to consider the Speenhamland system a fair test of guaranteed income as an alternative to the worthiness testing that is central to the Prussian welfare state.

Tainted or not, the idea of a guaranteed income has never died. Substituting a means test for a test of worthiness is a muse for those of us who contemplate the fate of the disabled worker today. The idea of a "guaranteed income" found advocacy in the United States as an alternative in "The War on Poverty," the cornerstone of the Johnson administration's Great Society and the Nixon administration's plan for welfare reform (C. Murray, "Looking Back," *Wilson Quarterly* [1984]: 97–139).

It resurfaced under the guise of a "negative income tax." In spite of his rhetoric advocating reducing welfare and increasing "workfare," Nixon tried to marshal a Family Assistance Plan through Congress. The plan entitled intact families with working adults to a guaranteed income supplement if their earnings were too low. The plan died in the birthing (D. P. Moynihan, *The Politics of a Guaranteed Income* [New York: Random House, 1973]).

However, the political process left behind two documents that inform the musings of all of us who wonder if a "guaranteed income" wouldn't provide a kinder, gentler, and more efficient and reasonable alternative for providing recourse for the poor than the current stratified worthiness testing.

One document was the report of the President's Commission on Income Maintenance Programs, delivered to the White House on November 12, 1969 (President's Commission on Income Maintenance Programs, *Poverty Amid Plenty: The American Paradox* [Washington, D.C.: U.S. Government Printing Office, 1969]).

This was a remarkable exercise, undertaken by an even more remarkable group of people, which included such titans of industry as IBM's Thomas J. Watson Jr. and Henry S. Rowen of the Rand Corporation. The commission concluded that an income-maintenance program similar to that in the Family Assistance Plan was more than defensible; it was overdue. Nonetheless, the moderates and conservatives were relentlessly opposed on the grounds that such a program would compromise "work ethic"—the Speenhamland legacy. In response to this debate, the Office of Economic Opportunity undertook one of the most ambitious social-science experiments in history. By that I mean a scientific experiment, not simply empiricism. The Negative Income Tax (NIT) experiment began in 1968, lasted for a decade, and recruited almost 9,000 subjects in sites in New Jersey, Pennsylvania, Iowa, North Carolina, Indiana, Washington, and Colorado. At each site, a sample of low-income individuals was randomly allocated to an experimental group that received income maintenance and a control group that did not. Economists have been mining this data set ever since. For our purposes, any and all who believe that income maintenance is a salutary and beneficent alternative to a stratified welfare state need to take note. Income maintenance proved counterproductive in that it reduced the work effort of the poor, particularly that of young males who were not yet heads of families. The results of the Seattle and Denver experiment are disturbing in that even marriage dissolution rates escalated (Office of Income Security Policy, "Overview of the Final Report of the Seattle-Denver Income Maintenance Experiment," May 1983 [⟨http://aspe.hhs.gov/hsp/SIME-DIME83/index.htm⟩]).

The outcome measures were short on assessing happiness. Maybe guaranteed income facilitated a life with more satisfactions than awaited those that spent their time shifting between poverty, working poor, and the pursuit of the dole. Even if that were the case, negative income tax as effected in the NIT experiment is no more than the lesser of two evils.

There still are scholars and politicians who seek a solution in income-maintenance programs. Many have rallied to the concept of a "citizen's dividend" to avoid any negative connotation of a "negative income tax." The idea is that successful nations are like successful publicly held corporations, only that all citizens hold stock as a birthright. Why not share the profits accordingly? One can find advocacy for a "social wage" in the writings of Thomas Paine, Martin Luther King Jr., James Tobin, Paul Samuelson, John Kenneth Galbraith, and many others at various points in their careers. Even today there are economists and political scientists of like proclivity. Since the worthiness-based system has weathered the last century very poorly, I suspect we will soon see a reinvigoration of the debate on citizen's dividends.

TABLE 8. Disability Awards under Workers' Compensation

CLINICAL DETERMINATIONS	CRITERIA
Causation	Injured? In the course of employment?
Consolidation ("Fixed and Stable")	Can more healing be expected?
Disability	How much work is left in the worker?

Bismarck did not turn to the Prussian medical establishment while designing his disability-insurance scheme. He did turn to physicians for help in its administration, however. Prussian medicine at the time was considered the pinnacle of Western medicine. The establishment was dominated by very reductionistic thinkers. For example, Theodor Billroth, a professor of surgery in Berlin, could declare, "If the whole of Social Medicine must needs be part of the curriculum of the medical student, it must not take more than two hours per semester, let us say, during the last two semesters; otherwise it will surely be detrimental to his other studies."[14] The notion that the physician was valued foremost for the detail in which he understood the diseases that afflict body parts is Prussian medical reductionism. Its legacy is alive today. It was this perspective that was brought to the issues raised in the administration of the Prussian disability-insurance scheme (Table 8). To qualify for workmen's compensation ("workers' compensation" in today's nomenclature), the inability to work had to result from an injury on the job. For Prussian medicine this was obvious: an accident is an accident, and an injury is an injury. Likewise, to imagine that a Prussian doctor could not determine when a patient had reached maximum medical improvement ("consolidation" is the European rubric) was insulting. As for the determination of how much work is left in a man, the Prussian answer, its ramifications, and its legacy will occupy us in the next chapter. In this chapter, the first question is our target.

The American Disability-Insurance Scheme

The United States has participated reluctantly and piecemeal in a dialectic that has yet to fully play out (Table 9). In the early decades of the twentieth century, "workmen's compensation insurance" made landfall, but not as a national program; each state legislated a version in its fashion and in its time. Prominent "social progressive" academics such as John Commons of the University of Wisconsin and Henry Seager of Columbia University,

TABLE 9. The U.S. Disability-Insurance Scheme

LEVEL OF WORTHINESS	INSURANCE FUND	INDEMNIFICATION
Work incapacity consequent to a work-related injury	Workers' compensation insurance	Wage replacement. Medical care related to the injury.
Work incapacity not consequent to a work-related injury in a worker	Social Security Disability Insurance	Modest pension if deemed incapable of earning minimum wage. Medicare for health insurance.
Work incapacity in someone who is not gainfully employed	Supplemental Security Income	Subsistence if deemed incapable of earning minimum wage. Medicaid for health insurance.

who founded the American Association for Labor Legislation (AALL) in 1906, called for a more comprehensive indemnity scheme. I. M. Rubinow, a physician and the chief actuary for the Metropolitan Life Insurance Company, became a leading advocate for social insurance,[15] particularly health insurance, to break the "vicious cycle" of disease and destitution.[16] In large measure, it is because of the AALL that workmen's compensation gained purchase. Congress felt that such a program would be an unconstitutional form of taxation. The New York State statute passed muster with the Supreme Court, however, and other states followed, one by one, over the next two decades. But neither the AALL nor Theodore Roosevelt and the Progressive Party could move Congress to accept a broader program of social insurance. Even the American Medical Association, in an altruistic moment, came into the fold, but to no avail. Woodrow Wilson's ascendancy to the White House signaled a pause in activity on this question that would last two decades. In 1934 Rubinow was still decrying "accident, illness, old age, loss of a job . . . the Four Horsemen that ride roughshod over lives and fortunes of millions of wage workers."[17]

With the Great Depression, the federal government's attitude toward these horsemen modulated a bit. President Franklin D. Roosevelt stood before Congress on June 9, 1934, and demanded "some safeguard against misfortunes which cannot be wholly eliminated in this man-made world of ours. . . . I am looking for a sound means which I can recommend to provide at once security against several of the great disturbing factors in life—especially those related to unemployment and old age." Roosevelt brought Edwin E. Witte to Washington from the University of Wisconsin to chair a committee to formulate the "sound means."[18] The Witte Committee, with such luminaries as Frances Perkins and Frank Porter Graham, was up to the task,[19] but the politics of the day could countenance only an old-age pension program, the Social Security Act of 1935. Disability insurance was mired in the argument that without a "strict test," there was no "safeguard" against unjustified claims. We shall return to this dialectic in the next chapter.

The Invention of the Regional Back "Injury"

All workers' compensation schemes in the United States are "no fault," meaning the employer is spared from personal-injury suit (tort immunity) with certain exceptions, such as evidence that the injury was intentionally inflicted. These schemes pay medical costs and lost wages consequent to personal injuries that "arise out of and in the course of employment," the language of most statutes.[20] The intent is to minimize the financial toll that compounds such injuries. In the early days, "schedules" were drafted stipulating the compensation for the loss of an eye, or a limb, or a life. When it became clear that workers could be harmed by more than physical force, such as by mercury and lead exposure or by anthrax, new legislation provided a remedy for occupational diseases. Even so, the notion of "injury" was contentious from the outset, as was the inflexibility of the "schedules."[21]

"Writer's cramp" and "telegraphist's wrist" were rallying cries of the early union movement in Britain, with the result that they were added to the British schedule for occupational diseases in 1908, but not without medical debate that culminated a decade later in the rubric "occupational neurosis."[22] If you first notice your inguinal hernia at work, is that a compensable injury? It became so when "rupture" became common parlance. As discussed in chapter 1, "railway spine" was a socially constructed affliction of passengers, not workers.

Regional back pain was not considered an injury until the mid-1930s, when W. J. Mixter, a senior neurosurgeon working at the Massachusetts General Hospital, ascribed cauda equina syndrome,[23] if not all backaches,[24] to disc herniation and described a surgical remedy. In the titles of his seminal contributions (cowritten with junior authors J. S. Barr and J. B. Ayer),

Mixter chose to term the pathobiology a discal "rupture," symbolizing the rending of normal structure. "Rupture" captured the attention of all workers' compensation administrators and adjudicators, as well as others involved in workplace safety and in the provision of remedies when safeguards failed. If the outcome is a "rupture," even if precipitated by an activity that is customary and customarily comfortable, the worker has suffered a compensable back "injury."

This inference informs our suffering and tests our coping with our next episode of back pain. Not only do we cope with the pain; we also cope with the notion of trauma. That is why our narrative of distress for backache can include the idiom, "I injured my back." That is why we physicians feel compelled to query a patient presenting with backache: "What were you doing when it started?" It is hard to imagine a similar exchange over a headache, absent some forceful trauma. Yet for seventy years the idea of back "injury" has troubled the lives of workers with disabling backache for whom workers' compensation insurance is designed to provide a remedy. Over the past few decades, the construct, the diagnosis, and many of its ramifications have been put to the test. We have learned why discal "rupture" is a flawed pathogenetic theory and compensable back "injury" a sophism that can make people sicker. These are object lessons that can inform social reformation.

As I have developed in detail in prior chapters, regional back pain has little if anything to do with ruptured discs or any other form of spinal pathology. The specific causes of regional back pain continue to elude scientific inquiry. Degenerative changes in the spine escalate with each passing decade until they are ubiquitous, but they have almost nothing to do with what we do in life. The age of onset and the degree of change are largely genetically determined; the contributions of environmental influences are barely discernible.[25] Our aging spines, however hoary, do not bear witness to a life of damaging trauma, nor do they offer anatomical clues as to the cause of our backache. They mark longevity, not decrepitude.[26] Back "injury" is a social construction, not a valid clinical diagnosis.

Traumatic amputations, fractures, and crush injuries can "arise out of and in the course of working." The "common cold" can also arise in the course of working, especially since so much of our exposure to droplet infections occurs in the workplace. But we don't consider the common cold an injury or even an occupational disease, although it may well be a transiently disabling illness. Certainly regional backache can occur in the course of working. But can backache also "arise out of the course of working," as an injury? Can biomechanical stressors that are usually comfortable turn pathogenic?

That seems intuitively appealing. After all, regional back pain is always mechanical; it hurts more when we add biomechanical strain to the hurting back simply by leaning forward. Tasks that were always comfortable at work and at home can become more daunting, if not prohibitive. The "back injury" construct holds that the physical demands that exacerbate the pain are the proximate cause of putative damage rather than an influence on the degree of discomfort. We need to liberate our medical and social welfare systems from this damaging misconception.

The Cochrane Collaboration reviewed multiple cohort studies in the contemporary workplace looking for some clue that a decrease in lifting and other materials-handling tasks would diminish the incidence or severity of backache at work. The collaboration concluded:

> There is moderate evidence that MMH (Manual Materials Handling) advice and training are no more effective at preventing back pain or back pain-related disability than no intervention (four studies) or minor advice (one study). There is limited evidence that MMH advice and training are no more effective than physical exercise of back belt use in preventing back pain (three studies), and that MMH advice plus assistive devices are not more effective than MMH advice alone (one study) or no intervention (one study) in preventing back pain or related disability.[27]

As is true of spinal pathoanatomy, the incidence of backache has almost nothing to do with the putative "minor trauma" of lifting tasks.[28] It is no surprise that the incidence of back "injury" has proved refractory to successive waves of ergonomic advice and devices, of clinical and rehabilitative inventiveness, and of regulatory and legal machinations.[29] Back "injury" remains the bane of the workforce despite the fact that the tasks in the modern workplace are far less physically demanding than those of earlier generations. And back "injury" accounts for the majority of the cost of workers' compensation indemnity schemes,[30] and workers' compensation costs consume 2 to 4 percent of the gross earnings of American employers.[31] We have known for decades that we were missing something, but the response was to fine-tune rather than alter our approach.

Ergonomics, Psychophysics . . . and Metaphysics

The invention of the "ruptured disc" and its coddling by workers' compensation administrators set the stage. But ergonomists and union activists conspired to entrench three ideas: a disabling backache at work is the result of the physical demands of tasks; a disabling backache is a compensable injury; and workplace safety considerations mandate appropriate modifications of the physical demands of tasks.

Ergonomics is a branch of industrial engineering. In the United States, it came into being to study the interaction of man and machine with a view toward efficiency. Ergonomists focused on time-motion analyses, looking for wasted motions and efforts. For this activity, ergonomics garnered little affection from organized labor. More importantly, it fell to ergonomists to suggest modifications of machines that would promote efficiency and effectiveness by the operator. Ergonomists are involved in the design of airplane cockpits, military conveyances, and much else to assure that an average operator can manage effectively.

Starting in the 1960s, ergonomists such as Erwin Tichauer added considerations of the comfort of the task to the efficiency and effectiveness with which it can be accomplished.[32] Tichauer took into consideration design parameters such as the shape and length of handles. He is the one who realized that a bent pliers was more comfortable to grip than a straight tool. Stover Snook pioneered "psychophysics" while working as a scientist at the research laboratories supported by Liberty Mutual, an insurance company that was formed in the legislation that brought workers' compensation to Massachusetts in the early twentieth century. Psychophysics is the study of aspects of a task that a worker finds more acceptable, aspects that vary from biomechanical considerations to ambient temperature.[33] These threads in ergonomics were of obvious value and found ready acceptance.

In the early 1970s, ergonomics made a conceptual leap that took it from the obscurity of utility into the bright light of importance. If a task is uncomfortable, some ergonomists reasoned, perhaps it is damaging. If Don Chaffin and his colleagues in the ergonomics group at the University of Michigan had doubts, those doubts vanished with the publication of studies that seemed to show that a mismatch between the strength of a worker and the physical demands of lifting tasks had something to do with back problems.[34] From the perspective of epidemiology, these were highly inadequate studies even in their day: definitions of outcomes, controls, and data analysis were unacceptable. To be charitable, these were ergonomists who were venturing into epidemiology. But they overlooked their methodological shortcomings and interpreted their studies as supporting their premise that uncomfortable tasks do damage to the low back.

Certainly if a task is unacceptable or uncomfortable, it should be altered if possible or shared or mechanized. However, if the task is customary and customarily comfortable and only uncomfortable when one has regional low back pain, does it follow that the task harmed the back and therefore should be altered in architecture or participation, if not eliminated? Modern ergonomics argued that it should be. Organized labor rallied around the conclusion of these ergonomists and remains steadfast in its support to this day. Organized labor is not wont to applaud the elimination of tasks either through outsourcing or mechanization. However, organized labor is adamant that tasks that are more difficult when one has a backache must be modified either by changing the task itself or by increasing the number of workers performing it. The ergonomic hypothesis has been a battleground in labor-management negotiations ever since these early studies. Furthermore, it has offered the plaintiff's bar new avenues for "toxic tort" suits, suits brought against manufacturers of putatively harmful machines. Several lifting guidelines have been promulgated by unions and even the National Institute of Occupational Safety and Health (NIOSH); the major guides lack consistency and validity in cross-sectional field studies.[35] The Occupational Safety and Health Administration (OSHA) participates in the fray by wielding citations and levying penalties on employers under the General Duty Clause of the Occupational Safety and Health Act.[36] This clause is meant to facilitate regulatory authority when a workplace is patently hazardous even if the hazard has not yet been stipulated in existing regulations. OSHA accepted the ergonomic hypothesis as its rationale despite the tenuous nature of the science. And, as we will discuss below, there was a concerted effort to establish ergonomic regulations in the Clinton administration, an effort that continues with some vigor today.

When occupational medicine was seeking firm footing as a discipline, its leadership decided that a master's degree in public health (M.P.H.) was to be prerequisite to board certification. M.P.H. degree programs were designed and offered at the Universities of Michigan and Cincinnati to accommodate these practitioners, many as part-time students while employed in industry. All were taught the ergonomic creed and most accepted it, planting it firmly in the core curriculum of their discipline.

From the 1970s well into the 1990s, ergonomists and their colleagues produced great numbers of observational studies probing for an association between the physical demands of tasks and the likelihood that a worker would find the next backache so intolerable that a workers' compensation claim for a back "injury" resulted. Associations were dissected out of these data sets, minor associations that were remarkably inconsistent. For all those who wanted the ergonomic hypothesis to stand on scientific footing, this literature offered volumes. There were those of us who were quick and visible in pointing out that this was volumes of marginal science and that there was a far more informative science. Nonetheless, NIOSH undertook an analysis that stands as one of the best examples of the fashion in which science can be perverted to serve a policy agenda. In 1997 NIOSH published its "critical review of epidemiological evidence for work-related musculoskeletal disorders."[37] This tome is a compendium of observational studies, stratified by body part, weighted by quality, and analyzed as to the strength of the association between physical demands of tasks and "injury." Chapter 6 is ninety-six pages of analysis of the observational data relating to the report of regional low back pain as "injury." Chapter 7 is sixteen pages devoted to "psychosocial factors," pointing out that while there is a literature suggesting these factors may play a role in the likelihood that workers would report a musculoskeletal disorder, the authors felt that there were "difficulties in determining the relative importance of the physical and psychosocial factors." As a result, the authors could justify not attempting to do so. In fact, there was abundant information on this point by the mid-1990s and the information has grown apace.

Back "Injury" as a Surrogate Complaint

Modern science has probed for and discerned associations with disabling backache that supersede the "injury" paradigm.[38] These factors even relate to the rate and degree of recovery from posttraumatic as well as regional back pain.[39] The result is an entirely different conception of the experience of disabling regional backache. As we have discussed, backache is an intermittent and recurring predicament of life. If you are a perfectly well, working-age adult, it is abnormal for you to make it one year without at least one important episode of low back pain. For many, backache is memorable;[40] for many more it resolves and is soon forgotten. Most of those who seek care, including medical care, heal rapidly whether they seek care in the context of work or not.[41] Recovery is an individual construct; for some, absence of pain outweighs improvement in function, and for others, the reverse holds.[42] After recovering from an acute episode, recurrence is unpredictable and far from inevitable; less than a third will experience memorable recurrences in the next year.[43] Some, a substantial minority, heal slowly if at all. For these, overcoming the challenges imposed by backache colors each day. Performance at work may be so limited that the worker sees no option but to seek a disability award under workers' compensation if the backache can be viewed as an "injury."

Common sense would indicate that the reasons one is more likely to find backache memorable or worthy of seeking care or disabling relates to the intensity of the pain, the physical demands of tasks, or the effectiveness of health-care interventions, but in this case common sense would be wrong. Alexander Magora was the first to understand this over thirty years ago.[44] His message resonated with few early on.[45] By the time we entered the twenty-first century, we were armed with an extensive and compelling science supporting the premise that confounders to coping with backache lurk in the psychosocial context of work,[46] and these confounders are far more consistently associated with disabling backache than those associated with the physical demands of work tasks. More recent studies from Manchester,[47] Brussels,[48] London,[49] Leiden,[50] Helsinki,[51] Copenhagen,[52] Washington, D.C.,[53] and elsewhere bolster this finding. A study by J. H. Andersen, J. P. Haahr, and P. Frost is illustrative.[54] They followed 5,604 Danish workers for two years, the great majority of whom experienced musculoskeletal pain, mainly backache. However, the transition from no pain or minor pain to more severe pain was influenced largely by psychosocial workplace factors, together with individual and other health-related factors.

The conclusions of the 2007 Cochrane Review mentioned above were reiterated in more recent systematic reviews of the world's literature from Australia[55] and by the Musculoskeletal Disorders Group of the Finnish Institute of Occupational Health.[56] The Finnish institute's conclusion: "There is no evidence to support use of advice or training in working techniques with or without lifting equipment for preventing back pain or consequent disability. The findings challenge current widespread practice of advising workers on correct lifting technique." In Europe, where ergonomics views itself as a "human factors" engineering discipline, these insights rest much more easily than in the United States, where ergonomics seems more fixed on biomechanics. Nonetheless, even the "Ergonomics Working Group" of

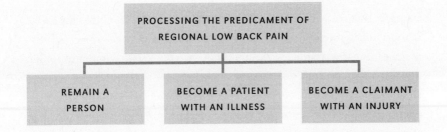

FIGURE 7. These pathways are the principal alternatives for the person with a regional backache. The fate of the minority is persistent back pain that precludes gainful employment. There are two programs that are designed to provide financial assistance to nearly all American workers who find themselves in such a circumstance. One is operated by the Social Security system and the other by the various workers' compensation indemnity schemes. Both rely to an important degree on physicians as gatekeepers. Both are tortuous but very different pathways. This chapter examines the interface between these systems and the claimants with persistent regional backache who seek disability awards.

the U.S. Department of Defense has recognized that "both work-related and non-occupational (psychosocial and others) sources of exposure" need to be considered when analyzing the causes of disabling regional musculoskeletal disorders.[57] Still the back "injury" construct is entrenched; it supports and is supported by an enormous enterprise that can lobby for legislated mandates and that is unshaken by study after study impugning its validity.[58]

The convergence of Mixter's inferences regarding discal ruptures and the workers' compensation insurance scheme has transformed backache at work into a surrogate complaint. As we discussed earlier, whenever one has a backache, one is forced to choose among three courses of action (Figure 7). We could deal with it as best we can while contending with all the solicited and unsolicited advice that bombards us. If life is bleak outside work, we are more likely to seek advice from a physician or some of the available alternatives. If life at work is relentlessly daunting and we see no alternatives or are offered none by our employer,[59] the next backache might seem the proverbial "last straw"; it is an "injury." If no physician, employer, human-resource professional, or claims adjuster (or the worker himself) realizes that the backache is intolerable and disabling because the worker finds the job hateful, unsatisfying, or insecure; the supervisor is insensitive, hostile, or cruel; coworkers are antagonistic;[60] the worker feels undervalued or underpaid; or the worker is overburdened by personal baggage, that worker is likely to see no other way out.[61] "I injured my back" is the resulting semiotic.

Does it matter that back "injury" is often a surrogate complaint? After all, the backache can be disabling nonetheless—not because of what is lifted but whether or when it is to be lifted. We might countenance such a surrogate if the result of launching a workers' compensation claim was likely to help the worker who is hurting. As we will learn in the next chapter, though, the consequences of playing out the surrogate complaint as a workers' compensation claimant are unlikely to be to the worker's advantage. Money will be spent in the attempt to fix the "injured" spine, in demanding the worker prove that the "injury" is disabling, in attempting to teach the disabled worker that the "injury" is not disabling, and in blaming the worker for not returning to the work that was unpleasant, even abhorrent, in the first place. In the aggregate, these are great sums of money in an exercise that misses the forest for the trees. More important, the worker is at risk for increasing symptoms in the process. The workers' compensation system is spending the majority of its resources to provide the worker with a back "injury" treatment that is tinged by racial bias,[62] ineffective surgery,[63] and invalid, if not fatuous, determinations of residual disability.[64]

Certainly the developed world owes its workforce employment that is comfortable when workers are well and accommodating when they are ill, even ill with such predicaments of life as the next episode of disabling backache.[65] However, there is a far more important legacy from the twentieth century's saga of the back "injury." Even more important than a workplace that is comfortable when we are well and accommodating when we are ill is a workplace that appreciates our humanity: our need to be valued, our need to feel secure, our need for some autonomy, and our need to see a future. "Human capital" deserves no less.

EIGHT

The Straw That Broke the Camel's Back

So regional low back pain is an intermittent and recurring experience of normal living. Furthermore, there is no such thing as a trivial regional backache—every episode gives us pause. After all, every episode alters our customary biomechanics so that even leaning forward in a chair is uncomfortable to some degree, and tasks such as putting on shoes can be challenging. Therefore, every episode is a predicament. The word "predicament" is chosen carefully. It has no negative or positive overtones. Life has many predicaments; regional low back pain is one that can never be totally ignored. We must do something about it, and as we have seen, we have a number of options (Figure 8).

I call choosing among these options "processing" the predicament. We all do it, each in his or her fashion. Prior experience, our particular "common" sense, our painfulness and our anxiousness all figure into the way we process a predicament such as regional back pain. Many episodes are so transient that we don't have time to consider options. Some can be blindingly painful, forcing prompt choosing. However we do it, the majority of us cope so well on our own that the episode passes and is not memorable for long. We might alter our activities, voice a complaint to someone near or dear, and swallow an over-the-counter analgesic to tide us over but do little else.

Sometimes, though, our patience and personal resources are stressed so much that we seek outside help. Despite our collective common sense, there are compelling scientific data that when we choose to see a physician or an alternative provider for help with the symptom of pain or for the symptom of compromise in function, we are driven less by the intensity of the pain

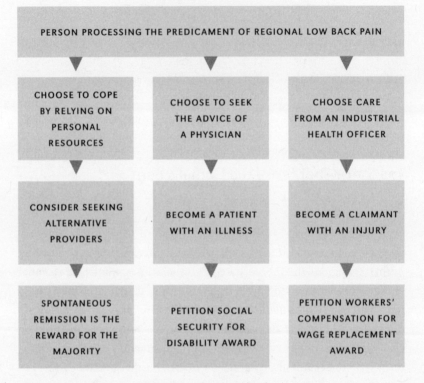

FIGURE 8. Processing the predicament of regional low back pain

and physical demands of living and more by the psychosocial factors in our lives that confound our ability to cope with this predicament.

In this chapter, we will consider the circumstance of persistent low back pain that interferes with the ability to maintain gainful employment. In the larger scheme of things, these are exceptional individuals. Given the ubiquity of the predicament, such exceptional individuals are not scarce in primary-care practices and certain specialty practices. When we did a household telephone survey in North Carolina in 1992, nearly 4 percent of adults described themselves as living with chronic low back pain; half of those thought they were in poor health, a third were permanently disabled, and most sought medical care frequently. Community surveys done elsewhere found similar results. When we repeated the survey in 2006, the number so afflicted had more than doubled. To my way of thinking, this is most likely a reflection of escalating unemployment in the manufacturing sector in North Carolina.[1]

We also undertook a cohort study in which we followed patients of over two hundred practices for more than a decade after their initial visit. Orthopedic, chiropractic, internal medicine, and health-maintenance-organization practices were represented. For the majority of people with regional low back pain who chose to seek care, the consequences were neither dramatic nor disheartening. Many different treatments were offered and accepted. Despite all these ministrations, nearly all felt well enough to return to being a person, most not worse off from this brush with largely ineffective interventions. I suspect most were changed forever by this interaction with the provider of choice, but that conclusion is based on my clinical observations and not on systematic data. We do know that patients are likely to return for treatment for recurrences, and generally to the same type of practitioner.[2] The care of some of the North Carolina cohort was indemnified by workers' compensation as a back "injury." Those who sought medical or chiropractic care as a workers' compensation claimant in the North Carolina cohort returned to functioning as quickly as those who sought care under some health insurance that was not based on their having been "injured." However, the workers' compensation claimant returned to prior life and workplace not so convinced that he or she was as well as before.[3]

The experience of patients in North Carolina is similar to that documented in cohort studies in other wealthy countries such as Britain,[4] Canada,[5] and the Netherlands.[6] However, the experience of workers' compensation claimants with acute regional back "injuries" in North Carolina, noted above, does not generalize as well. Much depends on the fashion in which the indemnity scheme is administered, the industrial climate, and other features that are peculiar to a given economy. For example, the Ontario Workplace Safety and Insurance Board is the principal provincial provider of workers' compensation, covering over two-thirds of all employees in Ontario. Workers who are out of work with an acute regional back "injury" in Ontario fare poorly; only 12 percent recover quickly.[7]

Compensating the Worker with a Compensable Regional Back "Injury"

It has been absolutely clear for over a decade that what or how you lift matters far less than whether or when you lift.[8] The notion of a regional low back "injury" is a fiction and any exposure criteria meaningless. That is why there is so much variability among workers' compensation schemes.

Some of these schemes attempt to quantify their definition of "injury" by attempting to weigh the contributions of the inherent susceptibility of the worker to low back pain (age, underlying spine disease, etc.) and the physical demands of the task being performed at the onset of the symptoms. Some are willing to consider the worker more likely to be injured if an arduous task has been performed over time, thereby invoking "wear and tear" (despite the contravening science). Some demand a sudden onset on the job. The AMA manages to countenance both the idea of injury and the attempt to assign,[9] but then the AMA would be risking much by doing otherwise—including a cash cow, its Guides to the Evaluation of Permanent Impairment, about which we will have more to say shortly.

All states mandate that employers purchase workers' compensation insurance for their employees. There is fine print in most statutes as to whether part-time employees must be covered or whether the mandate extends to employers with few employees. For all intents and purposes, workers' compensation is as close as we come to a national health-insurance scheme, albeit one that stipulates coverage only for employees and only when they are injured. Once "injured," the worker with disabling low back pain is entitled to all that money can buy to put it right.

Workers' compensation is an extremely efficient and cost-effective indemnity scheme for work-related traumatic accidents. If a worker suffers a crush injury, a burn, a laceration, or even death, whatever medical care and financial compensation are appropriate are provided expeditiously and without question. Furthermore, workers who have recovered from violent trauma tend to return to employment unless residual handicap is absolutely prohibitive, and they are usually welcomed back with open arms. The track record of successful management and reintegration into work life, however, pertains to traumatic injuries, not to compensable regional musculoskeletal disorders. Some 80 percent of claims relate to the former, but some 80 percent of medical and indemnity payouts relate to the 20 percent of claims that involve regional musculoskeletal disorders, regional low back "injury" in particular.

Workers' compensation programs in the fifty states, the District of Columbia, and the federal programs cost employers almost $90 billion but paid out only $55 billion in benefits in 2005. The difference is accounted for by administrative costs and the profits of the private companies that purvey insurance policies or administer programs for large employers who are self-insured. A few states, such as Ohio, Washington, and Oregon, have

TABLE 10. Defining a Compensable Regional Back "Injury"

CLINICAL DETERMINATIONS	CRITERIA
Causation	Injured in the course of employment
Maximum medical improvement	Fixed and stable
Disability	Impairment-based inference regarding wage replacement

government agencies that serve as the insurance purveyors and have been known to accrue enormous surpluses at times. For many years, the employers' costs for workers' compensation have risen faster than benefit payments for injured workers. The workers' compensation insurance industry is profitable. The cost to employers for the insurance averages 2 percent of wages but varies considerably depending on the "experience rating" of various sectors. Those with more claims, such as the construction industry, are charged more. Even in the construction industry, where traumatic claims are frequent, regional low back injuries are the most frequent claims and account for the greatest percentage of construction claim costs and disability days.[10] Of the total sum of benefits paid out, slightly less than half is for medical care and the remainder for cash benefits relating to wage replacement. The costs of medical treatments have continually escalated, accounting for the entire growth in benefit payments.[11]

Table 10 is a modification of Table 7 in the last chapter in which I discussed the medical determinations that were required in the administration of the Prussian social-insurance scheme. Table 10 is specific to the situation in the United States today. As discussed above, the idea that a regional backache could qualify as an "injury" has been embraced by the administrations of workers' compensation indemnity schemes. But the notion that a particular regional backache is an "injury" is often contested. An entire legal specialty is dedicated to assisting workers whose compensation claims for a regional back injury are met with administrative resistance. Typically, the legal fees are contingent upon the outcome of the claim; the attorney receives a percentage of the award if the claim is successful. It is the responsibility of the attorney to help the worker assert symptoms in detail and with forcefulness so that the claim is accepted and to garner fair compensation if there is residual disability when no further healing is deemed possible. As is true for any personal-injury tort, the process thwarts coping with the symptoms and discourages the plaintiff from perceiving improvement. There is even an inherent conflict of interest; the more the claimant improves, the less the award and therefore the contingency fee. Epidemiologists have probed the relationship between legal counsel and outcomes in workers' compensation data sets. The association with longer "patienthood" is consistent and strong.[12] The rejoinder is that the more severely "injured" are more likely to have legal counsel. If the experiences with tort reform for "whiplash"[13] are relevant, however, this rejoinder is very tenuous.

The Contest of "Maximum Medical Improvement"

"Maximum medical improvement"—the determination that no further improvement is likely—is very much the purview of physicians, and not just the treating physicians, as we shall see. Every workers' compensation statute stipulates that the injured worker is entitled to all medical care necessary to the reemergence of the "whole man." Determining the degree to which healing falls short of rendering one "whole" again is the task of disability determination.

This entitlement is a double-edged sword for the worker with a compensable back "injury." That worker is not a *patient* with a regional back illness; he or she is a *claimant* with a regional-back-pain injury. We know that elements of job dissatisfaction are likely to be prominent drivers of the claim at the outset,[14] causing the worker to have an edge of resentment, even anger, in the complaining. Then again, this is not an anxious patient wondering why he or she is suffering with backache. This is a worker who, by virtue of being accepted as a workers' compensation claimant, is certified as having been injured on the job and by the job. As a consequence of the injury, pain in the low back is challenging his or her ability to work and thereby adding insult to injury. Questioning the degree to which the back is painful or the pain is disabling sounds like, and often is, a challenge to the worker's veracity. Furthermore, there is no way to objectively quantify the pain and no pathoanatomical change that can be reliably ascribed to exposure at work or be considered the specific cause of the pain.

Veracity is all the injured worker has to validate the claim. As I said years ago, "If you have to prove you are ill, you can't get well."[15] Being challenged naturally causes anyone to focus on his or her symptoms, to recall the waxing more than the waning of symptoms, to be less inventive in

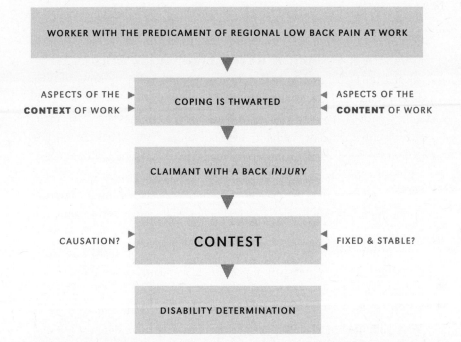

WORKER WITH THE PREDICAMENT OF REGIONAL LOW BACK PAIN AT WORK

ASPECTS OF THE
CONTEXT OF WORK

COPING IS THWARTED

ASPECTS OF THE
CONTENT OF WORK

CLAIMANT WITH A BACK *INJURY*

CAUSATION?

CONTEST

FIXED & STABLE?

DISABILITY DETERMINATION

FIGURE 9. The gauntlet to disability determination for the worker who has a compensable regional low back "injury" passes through a contest that can last many months if
not years. Since, by definition, regional back injuries occur in the course of performing
tasks that are familiar, customary, and customarily comfortable, a regional backache
is never labeled an "injury" without some administrative hesitancy if not inquisitive-
ness. The label never rests easily with human resources or workers' compensation
authorities. Since the claim is often launched out of and always with a degree of
resentment, administrative hesitancies are inflammatory. When it comes to medical
and surgical decisions, the claimant is at a far greater disadvantage than the patient.
Refusal of treatment taints the claimant with innuendo that he or she does not really
want to get well and return to work.

circumventing activities that might aggravate them, and to consider any
coincidental regional musculoskeletal disorder as yet another setback. At
the outset of the contest, the pain experienced by a worker with a regional
back "injury" is distressful and colored with elements of depression; elements of "fear avoidance" are acquired the more the claim is contested.[16]
In other words, the longer claimants have to prove they are hurting, the
more disabled they become by the fear that activity will hurt. *Patients* who
are receiving wise counsel are less likely to fall into these sinkholes; for
claimants, it is a minefield that predictably elicits adverse illness behaviors
(Figure 9).

We discussed illness behaviors in the context of fibromyalgia in chapter 3. The context under consideration here shares the need to prove one is ill. "Adverse illness behaviors" is a pejorative term today, but it shouldn't be. Adverse illness behaviors can include magnification of symptoms, peculiar descriptions of distress, posturing, and other behaviors that are not consonant with the pathophysiology of back pain, as well as the resentment and hostility that color claimant-physician interactions. The behaviors of a patient seeking a disability award for regional low back pain or compensation for regional back injury often fall into the category of adverse illness behaviors.[17] Over the past decade, there has been increasing recognition of the importance of properly assessing and managing pain. In 1995 the American Pain Society advocated taking a pain score as the "fifth vital sign." In 2000 the Joint Commission on Accreditation of Healthcare Organizations introduced new pain-management standards aimed at upholding patients' right to effective assessment and treatment of pain from admission to discharge.[18] These are important advances in the management of some painful clinical states, notably postoperative pain, dental pain, and cancer pain. But I am convinced it is a setback in the understanding of the plight of and the management of claimants with regional musculoskeletal disorders in general and compensable regional back injury in particular. Patients with chronic regional musculoskeletal disorders asked to score their pain have learned to do so in such global statements as "Today it is a 6 on a scale of 10."

They also acquire ways to express their distress that are peculiar to this clinical situation. For example, the oft-heard statement "I have a really high pain threshold" is but a denial that one is magnifying one's symptoms. I am the consulting rheumatologist to a large population of patients with rheumatoid arthritis and other chronic painful inflammatory arthritic conditions. The nurses staffing my clinic also staff the neighboring clinic, a pain clinic with many who suffer with chronic regional back injuries. A patient with rheumatoid arthritis has difficulty scoring pain. They respond with queries such as "Do you mean now, or this morning?" or "Do you mean my hands or my knees?" They have difficulty viewing themselves in terms of a pain score. The claimants with regional back injuries learn to have no such difficulty.

There are major consequences for the contest of maximum medical improvement (Figure 8) begging wider recognition. Maximum medical improvement is also termed "fixed and stable" in some states, or "consolidation" in Europe. Regardless of what it is called, the contest revolves around pain—both its reliability as a disabling symptom as discussed above and its suppression once it is assumed to be reliable. And the contest deprives the claimant of a primary role in medical/surgical decision making.

Prescribed Invalidity

Disability determination nearly always occurs with the claimant on leave from the workplace and receiving financial compensation—a Temporary Total Disability award—while under treatment. Typically, the patient is advised to avoid activities that are painful. Such advice can be palliative in the acute phase of regional back pain, although the appropriate advice is to get on with life as best you can. After a few weeks in the contest, the association of pain with activity is less clear,[19] and any advice other than getting on with life is not palliative. Several methods have been tried to encourage early return to activity, thereby aborting the contest. Some have been subjected to scientific scrutiny. Physical treatments such as graded activity regimens[20] and ergonomic interventions,[21] as well as educational efforts,[22] have proved inconsistent and not very effective. Two are object lessons.

Norway has a population of 4.3 million. It is a wealthy, relatively homogeneous, and highly progressive nation and has provided its citizenry with a comprehensive Social Security program for more than half a century. In the past decade, the Norwegian Royal Ministry of Health and Social Affairs has undertaken a reevaluation of the program. One aim of this initiative is to improve the disability-insurance scheme. Fortunately, the ministry has had the foresight to underwrite the clinical epidemiology to test the effectiveness of any reforms—before and after the fact. Norwegian workers who find their regional backache disabling can take sick leave without financial penalty. For the first two weeks, the cost is assumed by the employer, after which it is transferred to the National Insurance Administration. Approximately 85 percent return to work in the first two weeks,[23] an "iceberg" of morbidity that has largely escaped epidemiological radar in Norway and elsewhere. Most of the effort at reform focuses on the 15 percent of workers who have not returned to work by the end of the two weeks.[24] Approximately two-thirds of them will return to work by the end of two to three months, and approximately one-third never return to work.

A decade ago, the ministry instituted a program of "active sick leave," by which the National Insurance Administration would underwrite full wages for workers with disabling regional back pain who returned to modified duties at the workplace. There was no discernible effect on the likelihood of long-term disability.[25] So the ministry designed a multidisciplinary intervention to educate and reassure the worker. This effort culled a tiny percentage from those still disabled at two months who were otherwise destined for long-term disability.[26] Norwegian workers who take long-term sick leave for regional back injuries are people who have been transformed into insurance claimants. They are drawn from the population at risk for insurmountable regional backache in Norway, have multiple somatic symptoms, and are generally "tired and worn out."[27] They have been described as having a "syndrome" of "muscle pain located to the whole spine as well as to the legs and head and accompanying sleep problems, anxiety, sadness and depression."[28] We identified this population in our discussions in chapter 3 and elsewhere. For these people who live under a pall, "return to work" is too narrow a public-health goal and likely to promote adverse illness behaviors in those it seeks to help.

P. Loisel and his colleagues in Québec devised a "participatory ergonomics program" for the management of workers with back "injuries" who were claimants for a month or more. This "Sherbrooke Model" involved the formation of a collaborative group for each case of persistent regional back injury. The group was led by an ergonomist and included the injured worker, the worker's supervisor, and representatives of management and unions. After observing the worker's task, the group came up with a "specific ergonomic diagnosis" and gave precise recommendations to the employer. The injured worker was also enrolled in a school for back-care education (a "back school") and a multidisciplinary work-rehabilitation program for "work hardening." The Sherbrooke Model was subjected to a randomized controlled trial, randomizing forty workplaces to the model or to usual care.[29] Patients in the Sherbrooke Model group returned to work twice as fast; those in the model group remained out of work an average of 67 days versus 131 days for those in the referent group.

In the publication of this study, this impressive result was ascribed largely to the ergonomic intervention. Truth be told, a subsequent report published four years later revealed that most employers never followed the ergonomic prescription.[30] The Sherbrooke Model is in fact a convoluted form of mediation. Why anyone would still believe that the physical demands of tasks are the critical factor in disablement from regional low back pain is troubling. No one yet has been able to modify the physical demands of tasks to decrease disablement despite continued efforts.[31] It is not the task in the modern workplace that is limiting; it is the panoply of personal and other psychosocial factors that compromises coping with regional backache and thereby predisposes one to suffer the back pain as disabling and launch a workers' compensation claim.[32]

Opioid Analgesia

These claimants enter the contest with pain as their chief complaint. No claimant—and usually no physician, either—is inclined to hear this complaint as a surrogate for some other complaint. Most patients have sampled over-the-counter analgesics without medical encouragement and found them lacking. I have written elsewhere at length on the history, pharmacology, marketing, and abuses relating to prescription non-narcotic analgesics.[33] Here I wish to discuss the prescription of opiates in the setting of the contest of maximum medical improvement. None of the many treatment guidelines for low back pain countenances opiate analgesia. Yet opiates are commonly prescribed for claimants with disabling regional back pain and associated with poorer outcomes in this population.[34] The earlier opiates are prescribed, the more likely the claimant will not improve.[35] In the setting of chronic low back pain, opiates are not distinguishable from non-narcotic analgesics in terms of effectiveness[36] or lack of effectiveness.[37] Furthermore, in this setting, opiates are often associated with substance-abuse disorders.[38]

When will we ever learn? These claimants are victims of social iatrogenesis, a common sense that is harmful to their health. They are seduced into thinking that their regional low back pain is a disabling injury consequent to a workplace accident. They are forced to use the painfulness to validate their quest for indemnified health care and disability awards. Whatever psychosocial influences rendered their backache intolerable in the first place, the contest over these awards superimposes further suffering on the pain in their back. They are told their disablement will not resolve until their pain is squelched. They learn to think of themselves as a pain score. They embark on the Sisyphean task of treating their suffering with opiates that are said to be specific for pain yet seem too weak for the job, leading them to take escalating doses. They acquire increasingly maladaptive illness behaviors and elicit more and more disdain from most of the others involved in their care. No one tells them that opiates are ineffective for their pain and only confound their suffering. And this is just the beginning of their saga. Since neither time nor opiates are working, what do they have to lose by seeking a surgical remedy?

Surgical Zeal

I wonder how many patients would consent to surgery for regional low back pain if they had read chapter 6 of this book. Even for prolonged regional low back pain, there is no science to support a surgical option. Let me say that more correctly: there is a science that probed for benefit from surgery, but none was found. Therefore, the best current science proscribes surgical options. Elective procedures that have not withstood scientific testing should not be indemnified, and they would not be if it were not for the perverse nature of American health and workers' compensation insurance schemes. No sensible patient would accept a surgical intervention were it not for his or her preconceptions and misinformation, coupled with a surgeon's hubris. If the surgeon had to affirm that only his clinical judgment indicated that surgery was needed, many a patient would demur.

No claimant can demur so readily, if at all. To do so carries the implication that the claimant does not want to do everything possible to get well enough to return to work and thereby forgo the disability award. As a result, a lot of surgical procedures are performed on claimants, including a lot of innovative and repeat procedures. When claimants are not improved, particularly after multiple attempts, they earn the "failed back" designation, as if the failure is theirs rather than the flawed surgeries. And these surgeries do fail claimants many times more often than patients who are not seeking a disability award,[39] so often that one leading surgeon warns surgeons caring for workers with compensable regional back injuries "to be aware of this problem when advising patients and when analyzing results. . . . [B]e mindful of adding to the problem by reinforcing illness behaviour."[40]

Information about the numbers of claimants in the contest and their fate as it plays out is plentiful. The contest plays out in the United States with much more interventional zeal than elsewhere. We have very little information as to whether a long-term benefit accrues to the worker, however. There have been almost no studies of their fate once the case is closed. Twenty years ago, I petitioned the attorney general of the state of North Carolina for permission to do such a follow-up. It was likely that the Robert Wood Johnson Foundation would fund such an effort since studying workers' compensation was a programmatic priority at the time. Furthermore, I count among my colleagues on the faculty of the University of North Carolina leading and experienced epidemiologists, statisticians, and survey scientists. We could accomplish a follow-up study and maintain strict confidentiality for the workers in the process. The attorney general informed me, however, in no uncertain terms and in writing, that he would not sanction such a study and would consider it an illegal breach of claimant confidentiality if I were to go ahead. So I had to bide my time for nearly two decades, during which the peer-reviewed published literature describing outcomes following case closure for compensable regional back injuries remained scant. Then we had the good fortune to find a jurisdiction in Missouri where we were permitted to study a large cohort of workers' compensation claimants. My colleagues—Raymond Tait, John Chibnall, and Elena Andresen—and I were prepared to proceed and fortunate to gain the funding to do so from the federal Agency for Healthcare Research and Quality. I will say much more about our results shortly. The influence of surgery on the course of claimants in this Missouri study, however, is highly relevant to our current discussion.[41] This jurisdiction offered the opportunity to examine racial inequalities in the workers' compensation scheme. Whites were 40 percent more likely than African Americans to receive a diagnosis of a discal herniation. Furthermore, whites with this diagnosis were over twice as likely to undergo spine surgery. Since all were comparably indemnified, something else was influencing surgical decision making. African Americans in the cohort received lower disability ratings and settlement awards, but paradoxically they were spared unnecessary surgery.

Returning to work and terminating the claim aside, the contest of maximum medical improvement draws to a halt when the treating physicians can think of nothing else to do to the claimant or the claimant refuses to go along any more. At that point, the claimant is declared "fixed and stable" and moves on to disability determination, upon which a disability award is based. Before discussing disability determination, the workers' compensation system supports two additional experiences with which many a claimant will contend and that are worthy of our consideration.

Independent Medical Examinations

There is a difference between a consultation and an independent medical examination (IME). The consultant is chosen by the treating physician with the approval of the patient in the hope that the consultant can offer insights that will enhance the patient's care. The consultant becomes a treating physician, and a consultation becomes a collaboration. The IME is contracted by a third party to offer insights to that third party regarding the condition of the patient. The patient is usually a plaintiff or a claimant. The IME provides oversight, not treatment, which may involve only reviews of records or detailed examinations, including sundry laboratory tests.

No one performing an IME, however, should assume that the examination is exclusively for the benefit of the contracting agency. In 2004 the Michigan and Arizona Supreme Courts, followed by a number of others, stipulated that in serving the contracting agency, the examining physician cannot neglect duties to the person examined. There are duties to not cause harm, to diagnose accurately, to disclose findings to the person examined, and to maintain confidentiality.[42] I am hopeful that these judicial precedents will dramatically reel in the imperiousness of the IME. In many an arena, the IME's conclusions are an opinion based on the presuppositions and clinical judgment of the examiner, which can override whatever science is informative.

The IME function is contracted in settings not relevant to our considerations, such as in tort proceedings. However, the IME function is increasingly invoked by the insuring agency during the contest of maximum medical improvement, usually to question whether a diagnostic or therapeutic intervention is appropriate. The IME is also often invoked for disability determination under workers' compensation and by the Social Security Administration (SSA), where the IME is termed a "contracted examination." We will discuss those circumstances shortly.

It should come as no surprise that we have precious little information about IMEs other than they are often part of the contest for low back injuries and are often expensive. The examiners charge "customary" fees, which for surgeons may be as much as they'd charge for a comparable amount of time in the operating room. Performing IMEs can be lucrative. In the workers' compensation contest, IMEs are asked to opine as to the magnitude of the "injury" and the appropriateness of interventions. The former nearly always is an exercise in judging the veracity and character of the claimant. The quest for a specific diagnosis has usually played out already.

The IME typically is watchful for signs of feigning or symptom magnification. Suspicions can be raised if the findings on physical examination appear "non-physiologic."[43] For example, if the patient's pain is exacerbated when the hip is flexed while recumbent but not when the knee is extended while seated, one might be suspicious of adverse illness behavior, if not feigning, since both motions stretch the sciatic nerve. Psychological tests of memory and cognitive function have been used to probe the veracity of claimants with regional musculoskeletal injuries.[44] All of this makes me very uncomfortable with and quite critical of the IME process because, to my way of thinking, it promotes additional maladaptive illness behaviors. The beleaguered claimant already has enough of these as a consequence of the contest and whatever motivated the claim in the first place. Nonetheless, IMEs are an entrenched feature of the contest and are touted as enhancing the efficiency of processing the claim for a compensable regional back injury.[45] I never perform IMEs.

Pain and Work-Hardening Clinics

When the contest draws to a close, disability determination looms. The magnitude of the award reflects the quantity of disability, often captured as the degree to which the claimant falls short of returning to being "whole." These permanent partial awards can be lump-sum or long-term pensions. The insurance companies prefer the latter, as they have an actuarial business model; that is, they charge premiums so they can "bank" the amount they will need to cover the disability award until the worker reaches age sixty-five, and they are free to use these moneys for investments in the interim. The plaintiff's bar prefers lump sums to feed their contingency fees. The size of the award would diminish if the fixed and stable worker could return to the workforce in some capacity, particularly the prior capacity. That means that trying to further reduce the level of pain and begin to improve functional capacity would seem a fiscally sound goal were it not for the conflicting issues just mentioned. In fact, the attempts to help the worker regain functioning represent a very expensive undertaking with little yield.

The goal of pain reduction has led to the proliferation of pain clinics, often staffed by anesthesiologists willing to manage opioids, inject various parts of the body with local anesthetics and steroids, and even place spinal-cord stimulators. Despite the absence of compelling observational studies, let alone systematic studies,[46] all of these unproved remedies are underwritten by workers' compensation carriers. IMEs are generally of like mind. The needling is expensive. Few pain clinics claim much of a track record in returning people to work; theirs is more of a holding effort with hopes of slow improvement.

Work-hardening and multidisciplinary rehabilitation clinics take the opposite tack. Given the fact that invalidity persists despite all the interventions mentioned above, maybe the opposite approach would work. Taper off the opiates, get active and fit, and rethink options and outlook. Such a therapy program can last months, usually with many outpatient visits but occasionally in inpatient rehabilitation centers. It too is costly, often costing the insurer tens of thousands of dollars per claimant. Many of these facilities tout their track records in returning claimants to work. Some may have sufficient clout to drive that outcome. For example, they may be in a position to declare that if a claimant is not better in x months, it is a sign of their willful intransigence and disability rewards should be adjusted accordingly. The plaintiff's bar does not countenance such imperiousness often or for long.

There have been many, many randomized controlled trials of various forms of multidisciplinary rehabilitation and work-hardening programs. In the past decade, the Cochrane Collaboration and others have repeatedly taken a razor to the literature; the search for evidence of benefits is largely fruitless. The Cochrane Collaboration recently revisited the literature on back schools[47] and behavioral treatments.[48] The studies are inconsistent, and the evidence one can shake out is for effects that are far from robust. Various injection therapies[49] and transcutaneous electrical nerve stimulation[50] did not fare even that well. Attempts to find subsets of claimants in back schools or multidisciplinary rehabilitation programs who are helped by the experience are thwarted by the wide variety of the treatments and claimants and the inadequacy of the studies.[51] There is a suggestion of benefit from biopsychosocial rehabilitation[52] and other programs that focus on psychological issues,[53] particularly those emphasizing cognitive behavioral approaches.[54] At best, however, all of this effort results in an improved sense of well-being but not enough of an improvement to return to work, let alone to feel "whole" again. Furthermore, the most encouraging suggestions as to the effectiveness of multidisciplinary rehabilitation programs come from Europe. The contest in the United States is distinctive; it is infamously vicious in terms of litigiousness, surgical inventiveness, and the aggressiveness of the anesthesia-pain community. Claimants limp into the multidisciplinary clinics, having lost all hope and all self-efficacy, expecting the worst and fearing that almost anything they do will worsen the pain. Then they hear someone telling them that their pain isn't bad, get over it; inactivity is bad, get on with it; throw away your pills; and go back to the job that you found unsatisfying and unsatisfactory in the first place or move on to some lesser job. It's Kafkaesque. It is a drawn out, illness-inducing, painful preamble to disability determination.

Impairment-Based Disability Determination

After maximum medical improvement, how does one quantify how much work is left in the claimant? In the seventeenth century, Thomas Syden-ham taught us that symptoms were indicative of an underlying pathologic process and that logic dictates that treating the underlying process would result in the resolution of the symptoms.[55] Prussian medicine took this notion to great heights, which modern medicine maintains to this day in the "differential diagnoses," the probabilistic listing of diseases that could account for a patient's illness. On the occasions when this line of reasoning is productive, such as specific infections, the illness-disease paradigm is triumphant. The focus on the underlying disease largely neglects the illness experience. In chapter 2 we discussed how regional back pain is an example of the downfall of this mindset. For Prussian medicine, there was no downfall.

So when asked for a solution to the conundrum of disability determination a century ago, Prussian medicine put forth the converse of the illness-disease paradigm. If medicine was so good in deducing disease from symptoms, wouldn't it be effective in deducing illness from disease? The more disease found, the more one would expect illness. It follows that at some level, disease would compromise job performance and therefore account for the "illness" of work incapacity. In the realm of disability determination, the disease is termed "impairment" and the illness of work incapacity is termed "disability." In the early days of workers' compensation, "schedules" of impairments stipulated disability awards: so much for loss of an eye, more for loss of a hand than a foot, more for a thumb than the fifth digit, and so on. Of course, the flaws in impairment-based disability determination were obvious at the outset, even for loss of body parts. For a pianist, loss of the fifth digit is a major impairment, while it might not be so catastrophic if the task involved power gripping. For injuries where function was not lost but compromised, scheduling was no match and the process rapidly became confrontational.

The descent of the claimant into the nightmare of disability determination has much in common with Franz Kafka's bank clerk, Josef K., in *The Trial*, who is arrested but never informed of the charges against him. Reeling from his experience before the tribunal, he leaves the room and asks a person he knows to be familiar with such proceedings to enlighten him.[56]

> "Apparently you don't know the people there yet and you might
> take it up wrongly," his informant starts. "You must remember that
> in these proceedings things are always coming up for discussion
> that are simply beyond reason, people are too tired and distracted
> to think and so they take refuge in superstition. . . . And one of
> the superstitions is that you're supposed to tell from a man's face,
> especially the line of his lips, how his case is going to turn out.
> Well, people declared that judging from the expression of your lips
> you would be found guilty, and in the near future too."

Josef K. goes on to ask whether there is some commonality, some consensus, underlying adjudication, and his companion answers: "[T]hey have few interests in common. Occasionally a group believes it has found a common interest, but it soon finds out it's a mistake. Combined action against the Court is impossible. Each case is judged on its own merits, the Court is very conscientious about that, and so common action is out of the question." Josef K. is driven mad by the process.

Kafka was born in Prague in 1883 into a German-Jewish-Bohemian family. He received his doctorate in jurisprudence from the University Karls-Ferdinand in Prague in June 1906 and worked as a government functionary until his death at age forty-one from tuberculosis. During his lifetime, he published only a few short stories. *The Trial* and *The Castle* were published posthumously by Max Brod despite Kafka's expressed desire that Brod destroy the manuscripts. Brod, a prolific novelist, was Kafka's lifelong friend and law-school classmate. Brod, too, supported himself as a bureaucrat until he fled to Palestine ahead of the Nazi invasion. Brod also edited Kafka's diaries and explained the internal torment that motivated *The Trial*. From 1908 to 1913, Kafka worked in the Workers' Accident Insurance Institute for the Kingdom of Bohemia in Prague. Here is how Brod describes the impact of this experience with workers' compensation on Kafka:[57]

> It is clear that Kafka derived a great amount of his knowledge of
> the world and of life, as well as his skeptical pessimism, from his
> experiences in the office, from coming into contact with workmen

suffering under injustice, and for having to deal with the long-drawn-out process of official work, and from the stagnating life of files. Whole chapters of the novels *The Trial* and *The Castle* derive their outer covers, their realistic wrappings, from the atmosphere Kafka breathed in the Workers' Accident Institute.

It only took a decade for the Prussian formulation of impairment-based disability determination to turn Kafkaesque.

In the early decades of the twentieth century, state by state, the United States adopted the Prussian model for workers' compensation insurance—impairment-based disability determination and all. No such safety net was provided the worker whose disability could not be ascribed to a workplace accident in the Social Security Act of 1935. The consensus of committee after committee for the next two decades was that disability insurance was desirable, but management would be difficult and cost prohibitive unless some "safeguard" against unjustified claims of total disability, a "strict test," could be devised.[58]

Congressional committees favored the Prussian precedent of delegating the responsibility to perform impairment-based disability determination to physicians, but physicians balked. Leaders of major medical organizations argued before Congress that such a role was anathema,[59] a "destructive contradiction of a medical system that simultaneously certifies people as totally disabled and seeks to rehabilitate them. . . . [L]abeling a person as disabled could weaken motivation for recovery. . . . [I]ncome awards on the basis of disability would provide a financial disincentive to rehabilitation. . . . [C]ertifying a patient's disability for a government program would be in conflict with the physician's therapeutic relationship."

Congress decided that "real" disease could be reliably identified by physicians through clinical techniques that quantify impairment. Social Security Disability Insurance (SSDI) was enacted stipulating that the determination of total disability be impairment based. Furthermore, the Social Security Administration (SSA) set forth the process in a document, "Disability Evaluation under Social Security," which has changed little through many editions. It is now called the "Blue Book" and is available online (⟨http://www.ssa.gov/disability/professionals/bluebook/⟩). The meat of the "Blue Book" is its listing of impairments, similar to the schedules in the early administration of workers' compensation insurance. Listed are the impairments that, if present, represent the "strict test" for justifying an award for a total permanent disability. Here is the 2006 listing for disabling regional back pain:

1.04. *Disorders of the spine* (e.g., herniated nucleus pulposus, spinal arachnoiditis, spinal stenosis, osteoarthritis, degenerative disc disease, facet arthritis, vertebral fracture), resulting in compromise of a nerve root (including the cauda equina) or the spinal cord. With:

A. Evidence of nerve root compression characterized by neuro-anatomic distribution of pain, limitation of motion of the spine, motor loss (atrophy with associated muscle weakness or muscle weakness) accompanied by sensory or reflex loss and, if there is involvement of the lower back, positive straight-leg raising test (sitting and supine).

A stipulation such as this has been listed since the initiation of the program. It is an indefensible formulation for many reasons. No patient with persistent disabling regional low back pain who chose to petition for SSDI (Figure 7) would qualify, since evidence of "nerve root compression" is a prerequisite. In order to focus this monograph, I have not included discussions of sciatica and other forms of regional back disorders that involve the nerves to the legs. However, nearly all the issues we have discussed relevant to regional low back pain would pertain to the subset of regional back disorders with leg pain whose impairment is listed. For claimants with leg pain who are listed, disability determination hinges on their wage-earning capacity.

Claimants for SSDI with regional low back pain without leg pain are not listed. They will have to embark on a one-year journey between Scylla and Charybdis, during which they cannot be employed (if they are, they're not disabled) and are unlikely to have health insurance (unless a spouse has employment with a health-insurance benefit). Since regional low back pain is not listed in the "Blue Book," they will be turned down by the state Social Security agency and turned down again on appeal. It is likely they will undergo a contracted examination to determine if they have impairment(s) comparable to those listed. Unless they have coincident impairments, such as emphysema, the contracted examination will support the agency decision. After two denials, most of these claimants appeal before one of a thousand administrative law judges (ALJs). About half of these appeals are successful, particularly if the applicant hires an attorney, whose fees will be subtracted from the award. There is further recourse, but it is even more convoluted and rarely broached. The ALJ has far more leeway in disability determination, as testimony by the applicant and testimonials by interested parties in the applicant's community can supplement determinations of impairment. But the role of the ALJ is quite idiosyncratic; one is often reminded of Josef K.'s experience.

About a third of those who applied for SSDI in 2005 and a quarter of those who applied for Supplemental Security Income (SSI) in 2005 emerged from this tribulation with a pension. The distinctions between SSDI and SSI are presented in Table 9; to qualify for SSDI, one must have had a significant work history, but disability determination is shared by the programs. The success rate for those with just disabling low back pain was much smaller, unless they were deemed in the contracted examination to have one or more additional impairments synergizing with the back pain. That is the case for most who receive awards for any musculoskeletal impairment, unless the impairment resulted from failed surgery. Many years ago, I participated in the musculoskeletal panel convened by the SSA to revise the listing of impairments. I asked why a failed hip replacement was listed as a qualifying impairment, whereas when the hip was involved in a systemic rheumatic disorder such as rheumatoid arthritis it did not qualify. The result of my query was that the surgeons formed their own subpanel so that they could define the qualifying postoperative impairments, notably following spine surgery, without my queries.

Although analysis of the IME function has proved elusive, we have some data about the contracted examination. A number of years ago, we set out to probe the thinking of physicians who were performing several contracted examinations each year but were not "mass providers."[60] A number volunteered to serve as our subjects. They were each given a stack of cards with a vignette about a forty-year-old unemployed white male they were seeing for a contracted examination as part of his application for SSDI because of over a year of disabling low back pain. The purpose of a contracted examination is not to assess disability but to provide the SSA team (usually a doctor and a vocational rehabilitation counselor) with the data necessary to decide whether the applicant's impairments were comparable to those in the listing. However, the report can include the examiner's opinion as to the claimant's disability, and the interview is loaded with interactions to that end. Each vignette ended with the assertion that this man was capable

TABLE 11. Criteria for a Disability Award in the Social Security System

CLINICAL DETERMINATIONS	CRITERIA
Causation	Not relevant
Maximum medical improvement	Ill for at least 12 months, or less if not likely to ever improve
Disability	Impairment-based inference that incapable of any minimum wage activity because of a listed impairment or one deemed comparable to that which is listed

of light work, meaning that he would be denied benefits by the agency. Through the stack of cards, the vignettes varied in permutations of descriptors: two levels of pain, two of occupational history, and two of mobility; normal or abnormal X-rays or physical findings; and three levels of mobility. At the bottom of each card was a scale assessing the doctor's opinion as to whether he or she would be more or less certain the man was disabled despite the fact that he would be denied benefits because he was capable of light work. It turns out that the doctors were swayed by all the descriptors except pain. For example, the worse the exam or X-rays, the more certain the doctor was that this man really was disabled. But in the context of a contracted examination, the symptoms were not considered relevant. This is impairment-based disability determination in its purest form. It is consummate Prussian reductionism, the disease-illness paradigm. It is not, however, medicine, which always starts with the narrative of illness. In the setting of a contracted examination, these physicians are not performing as physicians; they are agents of the state.

The disability-insurance scheme operated by the SSA is a mother load of data for econometricians,[61] statisticians, and actuaries, including the many in the employ of the SSA whose annual update of the descriptive statistics is readily available online. For example, the descriptive statistics for 2006 can be accessed with this URL: ⟨http://www.ssa.gov/policy/docs /statcomps/di_asr/2006/index.html⟩. To qualify for SSDI, one must have been employed and contributing to the Social Security fund in at least five of the ten most recent years. The disability criteria are the same for SSDI and SSI (Table 11), and both are administered by state agencies. The

TABLE 12. Annual Social Security Disability-Insurance Awards for Musculoskeletal Impairments, Largely Disabling Regional Low Back Pain

ANNUAL SSDI AWARDS	1983	2003
Total number	41,782	199,014
Awards per 1,000 insured	0.39	1.38
Share of all awards	13.4	26.3

funding for SSDI is from the federal coffers; for SSI, it is from state coffers and varies in beneficence. About 80 percent of the nonelderly adults deemed disabled qualify for an SSDI award; the remainder qualifies for a disability award under SSI. In 1985 about 2 percent of adults were on the SSDI rolls; this doubled by 2005. The escalation reflects the fact that more and more people gain access to the rolls each year than leave because of death, retirement age, or recovery of work capacity. At the current rate of escalation, more than 6 percent of the eligible adult population will be on SSDI early in next decade if not sooner. In 2006 over 7 million Americans were on SSDI and over 3 million on SSI. The category of impairment that is associated with the greatest number on the rolls, the most rapid rise in award rate, and the most awards per year per insured is the "musculoskeletal disorders," with spinal disorders largely the common denominator. This is illustrated in Table 12.

It is difficult to imagine that this escalation reflects some erosion in the health of the American spine. It is easier to imagine that the psychosocial elements that predispose one to launch a workers' compensation claim for a regional back injury, or to seek care as a patient with a backache, or to take "sick leave" in Europe[62] or Japan[63] for backache, operate in the arena of long-term disability. Ours is an increasingly complex society that, having reached something of a zenith in the 1960s and 1970s, has been progressively devaluing human capital. More and more, people are finding their life courses challenging, so challenging that such predicaments as the next backache are more likely to prove "chronic" and disability schemes more likely to offer the only option. The majority of applicants for SSDI and SSI who are rejected do not return to the workforce.[64] Economists have juxtaposed unemployment data with SSA data, seeking to determine if these rejected applicants lack gainful employment because they can't work or because they can't find appealing work (harkening back to Henry Mayhew in Victorian times). The association between the number of applications for unemployment insurance and those for disability insurance suggests that a growing fraction of discouraged or displaced workers are seeking disability benefits.[65] The cost of SSDI and the health insurance that is its handmaiden is racing neck and neck with other "entitlement" programs for swallowing the entire gross national product.

I have pointed out that workers' compensation insurance was our first national health-insurance scheme, albeit only available to the injured worker to heal the injury. As originally constituted, SSDI was not really our second scheme. There was no health benefit in the initial legislation. If you were ill and had limited financial resources, you might have a caring physician attending to you for a pittance. The alternatives were the charity clinics operated by religious orders or municipal hospitals, as had been the case since the Middle Ages. If you needed hospitalization, there were the wards of municipal hospitals or the "teaching service" of academic centers. I witnessed all this as a youngster, a student, and a resident physician. The provision of a health benefit under SSDI had to wait for the passage of Medicare in the mid-1960s. The closest we came prior to that was the Technical Amendments of 1958, which permitted a taxpayer who was sixty-five and disabled to deduct up to $15,000 in medical expenses.

It is remarkable that even this came about in the 1950s. Arguably the most influential economist of that day was the Nobel laureate Friedrich Hayek, who was nurtured in the Vienna circle and moved on to a chair at the London School of Economics, where he was a colleague and friend of Karl Popper. Hayek was as powerful a political philosopher as the twentieth century would see. He was vitriolic when it came to socialism or anything that smacked of socialism because it placed the control of the economy in the hands of a few and predisposed to totalitarianism. His worldview bestowed rule of law on the state and the organization of society on the economy. For Hayek, socialist planning was unscientific and unnatural. He lived a long life (1899–1992) and was able to witness his philosophy drive the fear of communism of the postwar era and the free-market zeal of the Thatcher-Reagan era. It was because of Hayek that it seemed sensible for the nation to be alarmed when the AMA labeled national health insurance "socialized medicine." Hayek has had critics all along the way.[66] Few deny Hayek's influence on the development of social insurance in the United

States in the last half of the twentieth century, an influence that constrains innovation even today.

The Vortex of Disability Determination

Disability determination is not an objective process; it is a Procrustean bed for all but the most unfortunate Americans who suffer catastrophic disease or accident. Hidden under all the statistics and actuarial data is a human tragedy. The saga of the SSDI/SSI claimant with regional low back pain bears witness. I have long suspected that his or her fate pales next to that of the workers' compensation claimant with persisting regional low back "injury." As mentioned above, a Missouri workers' compensation jurisdiction allowed us to ask questions about the longer-term outcomes for claimants with disabling regional low back "injuries." Maybe this evil, wrong-minded, illness-inducing maze that masquerades as social insurance really advantages those workers who find their regional back pain intolerable and are drawn into the "exclusive" remedy that requires labeling their predicament an "injury." But as we have discovered, it doesn't—they are no better off. The impairment-based disability determination is totally unrelated to their function in the longer term.[67] Those whose permanent partial disability is deemed less important do the least well. They are mainly African American, dissatisfied with the workers' compensation process, poor, and poorly served by surgery. Their fate is to enter into the tortured labyrinth we call SSDI.[68]

The Medical Hegemony

My usage of "disease" and "illness" is in the tradition of Edward Huth, former editor of the *Annals of Internal Medicine*. He defined illness as the symptoms that brought one to the doctor and disease as what one has "on the way home from the doctor's office. Disease is something that an organ has; illness is something that a man has."[69]

As we have seen, in the early twentieth century, medicine assumed an expanded role as the arbiter of behaviors in society that were associated with particular *disease* states. Over time—and as medicine's "professional dominance" (Eliot Freidson)[70] and "cultural authority" (Paul Starr)[71] became ever more dogmatic—medicalizing work absenteeism and long-term disability came under the purview of physicians. Medicine's cultural hegemony continues unabated, despite dramatic changes in the organization of the U.S. medical industry. "Professional dominance" is largely in the hands of a small number of moral entrepreneurs, such as those responsible for the burgeoning of the cardiovascular enterprise, the corporate "academic health" center,[72] and the like. Medicalization grows more and more inventive, now encompassing kinship in the promise of genomics[73] and misery in the diagnosis of "fibromyalgia."[74] And disability has been balkanized so that the disabled are lost in a maze of process and definition.[75]

Reform is the topic of the next chapter. Reform is not a tweaking of the current system; that is window dressing. Regional low back pain offers object lessons: medicalization of life's predicaments, ineffectiveness of medical and alternative therapy, clinical and social iatrogenicity, and societal and financial barriers to effective therapy and to recourse for the illness of work incapacity. Today we are mired in notions that are long outdated and that can be informed by a robust modern science. Reform is not just long overdue; rational reform is feasible.

NINE

If You Don't Know Where You Are Going,
All Roads Will Get You There

Decrying the American "health-care system" has become an industry. Academics pick at it endlessly, politicians beat their chests, policy wonks are busy pitching quality and disparity fastballs, and administrators are leaping to "innovations" that impose the management strategies of the corporations on a human-services profession. Meanwhile, moral entrepreneurs are promoting health with tests that lead to no demonstrable clinical benefit and treating disease with interventions with questionable benefit, glossed-over risks, and ludicrous costs.[1] All the while, the print and broadcast media bombard us with an industry-supported cacophony of marketing that masquerades as health advice.[2] Speaking of which, the entire American institution of medicine is riven with financial conflicts of interest, from the "thought leaders" to the "academic health" centers.[3]

Who can doubt that the United States has constructed the most irrational health-care delivery system on the planet? In terms of health disparities, unconscionable benefit-cost ratios, expenditures that cripple the unsuspecting uninsured ill, treatments that are more harmful than helpful, and more, we have a system that is simply unsupportable. As we have seen, the treatment and fate of Americans with back problems is a poster child for this madness.[4]

There is a growing awareness in the population at large that something is dreadfully wrong with "health care" in America, that the programmatic tweakings and shufflings of moneys from pot to pot that are being advocated cannot be on the mark. Money cannot be the limiting factor: we spend over a trillion dollars annually, some 17 percent of our gross domestic product.

That's over twice the percentage spent by any other country, and for what? What value did we derive from the $30 billion we spent in 2005 on direct medical and surgical expenditures just for "back problems" (⟨http://www .meps.ahrq.gov/mepsweb/⟩)? Most of this has become painfully obvious to all of us, except maybe the overpricing. For example, for comparable drugs, the price per pill in the United States is 50 percent higher than in European Union countries. By 2006 we were spending about $450 per capita to administer our system, and no other country came close. France got away with $250 per capita, Canada was $150 per capita, and Denmark, Finland, and South Korea were under $100 per capita.

I do not want to belabor all of this shamefulness. That is not my style, nor is such a tack likely to be productive. The best we can do is to superimpose rationality on the current system—ironclad, science-supported, and patient-driven rationality with the goal of assuring health and providing recourse when that assurance falls short. We are advantaged by a cadre of physicians who are culled from the ranks of the best and the brightest and who would like nothing better than to do what is right by their patients. America seldom hears of them but, rest assured, they are there in numbers. I know, having been involved in educating and supporting so many for so long. They are our underground departments and silent majority who are rewarded more by gratitude, respect, and trust than by largesse.

Exploring the fashion in which American medicine falls short in general is the focus of two of my earlier books.[5] Here we are using regional low back pain as an object lesson that crosses boundaries of responsibility and entitlement in the contemporary welfare state in quest of a far more rational approach to promoting the welfare of the public. Two traditions in moral philosophy converged during the twentieth century to create the contemporary welfare state, one utilitarian and the other Kantian. The utilitarian is dedicated to doing what is pleasing to and valued by the greatest number. Kantian ethics values rational thought and personal responsibility over the acceptability of the consequences of our actions.[6] In the context of public health, the distinction is between concerns for sick people versus concerns for sick peoples. There is an inherent tension in this dichotomy, reflecting the degree to which there is dissonance between autonomy and paternalism, between the common good and that which benefits the individual, and between the result and the price paid in getting to that end. That tension has led to a communitarian ethic that imposes the shared values, ideals, and goals of the community—that is, the common good—on the wants and welfare of the individuals taken together. Designing a path up to this moral high ground is possible by taking advantage of twenty-first-century science.

The Health of the Public

There may be more nonagenarians today, but the percentage of the population that is reaching that age is not growing, at least not much, and most that arrive are decrepit. I am comfortable asserting that our species has a limit on life expectancy set in the near neighborhood of eighty-five years. If you are an octogenarian, it matters little which of the diseases that you have becomes your reaper; it is much more important that your passage is as gentle as your journey was memorable. If you make it to a ripe old age, does it matter what disease kills you? Life-course epidemiology is the science that informs the rules that govern the duration of the journey to all-cause mortality.[7] The proximate, or specific, cause of death is not relevant in octogenarians. What is accomplished if colons or breasts or prostates have been removed but the patient dies of something else at the same time? When we hear of "epidemics of fatal *xxx* disease"—heart disease or cancer, for example—we should learn to ask at what age; octogenarians die, and no one allows us to sign off on a death certificate with the diagnosis, "It was his/her time."[8]

We should be outraged when we hear of the elderly taking statins or oral hypoglycemics or subjected to invasive procedures for atherosclerotic conditions or regional back disorders. These are interventions that do not advantage the young; in the elderly, they can cause frailty or worse. The elderly deserve much better; they deserve attention to symptoms[9] and a caring community. The central challenge to the health of the public in a developed country is to get the people to age eighty-five in a journey that was satisfying and to assure that their dying is not lonely or painful. In this context, the health of the public hinges on the degree to which the people are comfortable in their socioeconomic status,[10] which is closely aligned with the composition of their residential neighborhood,[11] and the degree to which they are satisfied with their jobs.[12] Inadequacies in any of these life-course attributes place people at death's door in their seventies, not in their eighties; this is all-cause mortality. Furthermore, malignant influences in this context subsume nearly all the risk inherent in health-adverse behaviors and cardiovascular risk factors. That is one reason that programs to ameliorate such risks have dismal track records; the other is that the drugs used are ineffective and useless toward the end of life.[13] As we have seen, regional low back pain that is chronic, that causes one to seek care, or that is disabling is a window into this all-cause mortal hazard.

The Health of the People

Getting to age eighty-five in a satisfying journey is not a trivial challenge even for those who have the perquisite comfort in their socioeconomic status and satisfaction with work. For those without these advantages, life is not as long, but getting to their appointed hour is not a trivial challenge either. There are supervening clinical events for which modern medicine is often a match, such as trauma, appendicitis, some infectious diseases, and the like. There are diseases such as symptomatic coronary artery disease, rheumatoid arthritis, or multiple sclerosis for which medicine can offer benefits. In these circumstances, it is imperative that effective treatments be applied successfully and efficiently.

Then there are those many, many predicaments of life that cannot be wholly avoided and do not respond to treatment as disease; woefulness, heartache, fatigue, and grief are examples. These are not diseases but part of the life course of everyone. There are other ubiquitous morbid experiences that our culture is not wont to consider as predicaments of normal life course: headache, heartburn, sleeplessness, altered bowel habits, and many regional musculoskeletal disorders, to mention a few. These also do not respond to treatment as diseases because they are not diseases. Furthermore, all of these predicaments of life will be perceived quite differently if they are labeled "disease." Labeling them as such is called "medicalization." The labeling may be palliative, or not, and when not, it is likely to be iatrogenic, to lead to an increase in the intensity of the symptoms. Regional low back pain serves brilliantly as an example of iatrogenic medicalization.

The Enablement State

As Berkeley economist Neil Gilbert has so elegantly argued, the welfare state is undergoing rapid transformation into an enablement state.[14] This does not mean an end to social-welfare programs. Rather, contemporary economic considerations demand labor flexibility and the opening of new markets. In such a climate, social-welfare policies will increasingly be designed to enable more people to work to support the ever-expanding sphere of activity of the private sector.

I am no Luddite. I realize that the leanings of the liberally inclined and those of a more conservative bent are converging toward the formulations of Hayek, toward privatization, beneficent capitalism, and what Gilbert terms an "enabling state" that promotes working as a manifestation of solidarity. This dialectic is now the communitarian ethic. But speaking as a physician who has spent decades as a student of the illness of work incapacity, the primary goal of capitalism is not the accumulation of capital or even the opportunities that the accumulated capital offers; it is the creation of sustaining jobs. If the transformation from the welfare state to the enabling state does not value human capital, it will be doomed for the same reasons Hayek found socialism anathema. Human capital denotes more than a meritocracy. Valuing human capital requires a philosophy of life that tolerates lapses, empathizes with vicissitudes, and countenances failure. Valuing human capital recruits the mind of the poet as much as that of the economist. With this as my lantern, regional low back pain as the object lesson, and a good deal of humility, I will suggest a transformation from a welfare state to an enabling state that values human capital. For this transformation to stand a chance, some of the current fortress institutions need to be assaulted.

Putting the Health-Care Horse in Front of the Health-Care Cart

In the debates regarding health-care reform, one goal promoted by all is "quality." If medical professionals could only perform up to certain standards, the institution of American medicine would be supreme and vindicated. Unlike backache, myocardial infarction lends itself to a definition of the disease and of its outcome as well as to consensus as to its optimal management. That being the case, why is it that eliciting "quality" in the treatment of heart attacks with carrots and sticks does not improve outcome?[15] Those whose minds and mind-sets are fixed on improving quality argue that we must do what we are doing even better. I argue that what we are doing is useless at best and likely to be harmful. My argument is based on the literature that examines the effectiveness of what we do despite the theory—and the industry—that is committed to the current approach. The American approach to coronary artery disease is unsurpassed in terms of Type II Medical Malpractice, my term for doing the unnecessary even if it is done very well. The management of regional low back pain is another prime example, spine surgery in particular.

Quality of performance is not a goal in and of itself; it is only a goal if the performance benefits patients! The majority of the "health-care dollar" expended in the United States does not benefit patients. So many high-ticket items that are trumpeted as the triumphs of U.S. medicine are little more than a scam.[16] Spine surgery for regional low back pain has earned this ignominy. The first priority for reform in the care of the health of the American is to stop underwriting the profitably useless. We have the science to do so.

Evidence for Effectiveness

The science that informs utility hinges on the distinction between efficacy and effectiveness. Efficacy explores whether something works; effectiveness explores whether it works well enough to matter. The only compelling evidence for clinical efficacy, for an association between an exposure (a drug or device, for example) and a health effect, comes from randomized controlled trials.. Every other scientific research design is more susceptible to confounding, bias, and other distortions. These alternative research designs are called "observational studies." Cohort studies follow a group of subjects over time, relying on statistical modeling to seek associations with the development of particular outcomes. Case-control studies probe attributes of cases that might be lacking in people who are spared the particular health effect. Cross-sectional studies take a snapshot of a population at a given time and try to discern if those who have the health effect at issue differ from those who do not. All of these designs are far simpler and less costly than RCTs because they accept the subjects as they find them. But all have serious inherent shortcomings. Some of the shortcomings can be overcome by meticulous attention to the details of the study and analysis,[17] but no amount of maneuvering can overcome their inherent weaknesses. They are quick, down, and dirty ways to test a clinical hypothesis. If they are done as well as possible and there is no joy in the result, it is time to move on to another hypothesis. If the result is promising and you care, it is time to move on to an RCT. I am certainly not alone in my qualms about observational studies.[18] We are going to focus on the evidence of efficacy from RCTs in all of our policy considerations.

I discussed the difference between evidence for an effect (efficacy) and effectiveness in chapter 4. Evidence for efficacy offers one some degree of confidence that a particular association, say between a drug and a good clinical outcome in a particular clinical setting, is not likely to have occurred by chance. Effectiveness asks the crucial next question: given any particular instance of efficacy, do you really care? Is it evidence for an effect that is important enough, likely enough, and safe enough to be valuable to me?

If I told you that I had evidence that a statin, a drug that lowers cholesterol, prevented heart attacks, wouldn't you want to know the effectiveness? If I told you that I would have to treat 250 men with "high cholesterol" (but otherwise well) for five years to possibly spare one a heart attack but spare none death from heart disease, would you take the drug? How about if I had to treat only seventy for five years to accomplish as much; would you take the drug? How about if I told you that taking the drug would reduce your risk of a heart attack over the course of the next five years from 6 percent to 4 percent; would you take the drug? (I could also have told you that the reduction from 6 percent to 4 percent is a reduction of risk by 30 percent, a relative risk reduction, but that's an unconscionable mind game—unless I had also stated that the absolute risk reduction is 6 percent – 4 percent = 2 percent.) I have just presented the upper and lower limits of effectiveness of using statins for primary prevention of heart attacks based on the results for RCTs.[19] Statins spare 1 in 70 to 1 in 250 well men a heart attack over the course of five years and save no lives. I could have also said the absolute risk reduction is between 2 percent and 0.5 percent. Would you value this level of effectiveness enough to swallow a statin every day for five years or longer? Would you if you had to pay for it out of pocket? The usual definition of "value" in the health-care arena takes benefit, risk, and cost into account. For the moment, I will exclude cost from our considerations, but only for the moment.

I am belaboring the notion of effectiveness because it is crucial to the design of a rational health-care system. The public discussion of it has run the gamut from illuminating to obfuscating, a potential for confusion that marketing, and not just direct-to-consumer marketing, has learned to exploit. There has even been an elegant RCT of the different ways to describe effectiveness.[20] A large number of people were asked to place a value on a drug taken for five years to prevent heart attacks when the effectiveness was described in three different ways: postponement of a heart attack by two months for all patients treated, postponement by eight months for one in four patients, or sparing one in every thirteen patients from a heart attack. When the data on effectiveness was presented in the first format, 69 percent of the subjects said they would take the pill; in the second format, 82 percent consented; and in the last format, 93 percent consented.

Of course, all of these estimates of risk reduction are comparable. But in the last format, the "number needed to treat" (NNT) is most persuasive. Cognitive psychology suggests there are two influences on the way we comprehend risk.[21] We bring an analytic system to bear that takes advantage of whatever mathematical skills we can muster. We also bring a good deal of emotion to the table. The complex interplay between these two results in what for us is rational behavior. I am not sure whether being swayed by NNTs is the most rational of analytic choices, but it clearly resonates with most people's risk construct. I personally prefer knowing the actual data and deriving the absolute risk reduction. But a 2 percent absolute risk reduction implies an NNT of about fifty, and a 5 percent reduction is an NNT of about twenty. So the subjects in the RCT and I are in the same ballpark. Those of you who leap to "evidence" (efficacy) without discussing effectiveness are not on the same field.

Efficacy, not effectiveness, is the primary consideration in the studies of the Cochrane Collaboration, and it is the critical factor in licensing decisions for pharmaceuticals at the FDA. Evidence, not effectiveness, is the hypothesis tested in nearly all RCTs. Of all the organizations and agencies in the world of evidence-based medicine, only the American College of Physician's ACP Journal Club has been emphasizing effectiveness by the simple calculation of NNTs. Recently the U.S. Preventive Services Task Force has moved in this direction. There is a utilitarian rationale for accepting evidence for small degrees of effectiveness as persuasive, even determinative. The effectiveness may seem minimal, even trivial from the perspective of a given individual, but it may be sizable for the population at large. Hence, the NNT of 250 in the example above may spare a sizable number of people if millions are treated. Generalizing from an RCT to the population burden of disease follows from the pioneering work of G. Rose[22] but takes liberties I am not prepared to accept. It assumes that RCTs can be powered (in a statistical sense) to discern small effects reliably. As I detail in chapter 4, unavoidable and immeasurable error in the way subjects are randomized and much more should make everyone as wary as it makes me dismissive.

If we were to power trials for large degrees of efficacy based on some a priori consensus as to what is valuable, the size, duration, and cost of RCTs would decrease dramatically and their reproducibility would increase. Several such high-efficacy trials could probe for efficacy in subsets of patients—young, old, with confounders and without. We would no longer be studying tens of thousands of subjects for years in the hopes of being able to dredge evidence for some small effect out of the morass of data. Rather, efficacy of a high degree (a large effect) would translate into effectiveness for the subset studied.

The argument against efficient RCTs seeking such evidence for effectiveness relates to adverse effects. Such RCTs are unlikely to detect adverse effects that might be only moderately less frequent than the health effect being sought or that are frequent in subjects that might not have qualified for the RCT because they did not quite meet the criteria for entry (maybe they were too old or too young, had another disease, etc.). This is the "first, do no harm" argument,[23] and it is a telling one. However, RCTs for effectiveness offer an assessment of short-term, highly frequent adverse effects.

The only way to monitor for lesser and less-frequent events in a spectrum of exposed patients is with efficient postmarketing surveillance. This was one of many recommendations in the 2007 Institute of Medicine proposal for reforming the FDA and its regulatory role, to which the FDA has responded in part.[24] There is a proposal for a pilot surveillance program in the Veterans Health Administration system, a system that can readily capture drug prescribing and monitor clinical outcomes to the extent that the system is "single payer." The proposal for reform that I am leading up to in this chapter offers a much more global approach to pharmacosurveillance.

Devices, Procedures, and the Risk/Benefit Ratio

The third institution that we must confront is the industry supporting the design and manufacture of new medical devices. The Supreme Court decision in *Riegel v. Medtronic* removes the plaintiff's bar from the safety equation for devices, as we discussed in chapter 6. No doubt, there will still be suits relating to manufacturing flaws and operator errors, but the Supreme Court is assuming that licensure of a device by the FDA is prima facie reassurance as to safety; reassurance of efficacy is a secondary consideration, one that the FDA assigns in large part to operator judgment and competence. I wonder if the Supreme Court justices would have the same opinion if they had read chapter 6 of this book. On the other hand, the plaintiff's bar offers a very inefficient remedy. It is inefficient procedurally, since closure in one venue may mean little for another. Product-liability litigation is a difficult pill for the adjudicatory process when medical devices are at issue; the distinction between an adverse outcome and an adverse effect is seldom unequivocal in a given patient.

It is time for the FDA and the public in general to demand as much rigor in licensing indwelling devices for elective procedures as for pharmaceuticals. That means that scientific evidence for efficacy is a requisite for licensure. If there is a standard, tried-and-true device, there should be head-to-head RCTs demonstrating a meaningful reason to switch to the newer device and mandatory surveillance for adverse events once licensed. An example of this is the hardware for total hip replacements. We should never license an indwelling device if the result of the RCT is less than a meaningful improvement over the prevailing standard treatment; a result suggesting equivalence or "noninferiority" in the short term does not justify the uncertainties about problems in the future. I cannot countenance the innovation-for-innovation's-sake argument.[25]

I also am very wary of head-to-head trials. If there is a device (or a pharmaceutical) that is clearly effective, then it becomes the gold standard for treatment. RCTs would be designed to compare a novel approach with this gold standard. It would be unethical to compare the novel device with a placebo and thereby deprive the control group of a treatment known to treat their condition effectively. The choice to study the novel treatment head-to-head is as ethically demanding as the choice to give patients a placebo. Two questions must be answered before initiating a head-to-head trial: How "golden" is the gold standard? And how much more effective must the novel intervention be to supplant the gold standard? If the gold standard is barely effective, a demonstration that the novel intervention is equivalent offers a telling syllogism. If the gold standard is effective, how much more effective must the novel intervention be to justify exposing patients to unknown long-term risks?

The history of the introduction of surgical interventions for low back pain (chapter 6) is an object lesson. Since almost no intervention has proved efficacious, let alone effective, there is no interventional gold standard. There are standards of care that rely on consensus rather than science. And there are numerous examples of head-to-head trials comparing an investigator's technological brainstorm with the investigator's notion of standard of care. All the novel forms of disc removal, spine fusion, and disc replacement have been compared with the usual surgical procedure in head-to-head trials yielding equivocal results in terms of efficacy. Always the investigator declares the result a success because the procedure is no worse than the standard of care but stands on more sound theoretical footings—that is, the investigator's preconceptions.

Any suggestion that a placebo-controlled trial is necessary to establish efficacy is anathema on ethical grounds, as if the outcome were life or death. If it were life or death, the standard of care is the bare minimum one can do. But interventions for back pain are designed to provide relief of symptoms, less back pain, or improved function, and invasive interventions are even more prone to placebo effects (chapter 5) than pharmaceuticals or physical treatments. An RCT that compares an invasive procedure with a placebo that is less invasive introduces considerable bias toward the putative efficacy of the procedure. The only control that obviates this bias would be a sham procedure. There are precedents for sham-controlled RCTs of surgical procedures. The first and most dramatic comes from interventional cardiology.[26] There is a long history of surgical interventions for angina. In the 1950s the good idea was to tie off an artery, the internal mammary artery, which competed a little for blood flow to the outer heart muscle. It was thought that tying of the internal mammary artery would improve cardiac blood supply. The tying resulted in considerable improvement in these patients and much bravado in their surgeons. Then there was a double-blind, randomized, sham-controlled trial.[27] Neither the patients nor the people involved in assessing postoperative course knew whether the wound on the chest was only skin deep. It turned out that the patients did just as well with a skin incision as with ligation of the artery. The particular procedure died, the medical world gained cognizance of the power of the surgical placebo, and bioethicists have waxed eloquent ever since. It turns out the surgeons undertaking the trial did not inform their patients that they were being entered into an RCT. Would they have volunteered if informed?

Surgeons since have argued that performing a sham surgical procedure is harmful by its very nature and therefore presumptively unethical. The proposition of sham surgical controls has been a lightning rod ever since, with few willing to touch it in practice but many in theory. But those few have produced very telling results. One example is the sham-controlled trial of IDET, the probe discussed in chapter 6, which is inserted into the disc to heat it up. There have been a number of sham-controlled trials of injecting various spinal anatomical structures for low back pain; none of the treatments proved effective, nor did they when the comparator was noninvasive.[28] Another is a sham-controlled trial of arthroscopic surgery for painful osteoarthritis of the knee.[29] These subjects were fully informed about the nature of the trial. Slightly over half of the subjects eligible for the arthroscopic trial volunteered, which is a higher refusal rate than for most pharmaceutical RCTs, but not that much higher. I agree with the arguments of Franklin Miller, a bioethicist at the National Institutes of Health.[30] If there is no head-to-head alternative, if the risks of the sham procedure are minimized, if consent is truly informed, and if the risks are justified by the potential value of the science, sham-controlled RCTs are ethical. In fact, given the tragedy that is modern spine surgery and modern invasive cardiology,[31] licensing indwelling devices and condoning invasive procedures without scientific testing is unethical.

The standard for the licensure of indwelling devices or elective surgical procedures at the FDA should be the same as for novel pharmaceuticals. We, the professionals and the people, need to come to grips with the reason for stringency.

Patient-Oriented Clinimetrics and the Contract Research Organization

The last institution we will confront in this section is relatively new: the Contract Research Organization (CRO). A new drug application (NDA) to the FDA is a hefty document. At its core is the analysis of at least one RCT, which purports statistically significant evidence that the drug is as good if not better than any alternative drug. The licensing process involves convincing the FDA that this assertion of evidence is tenable and the need for the agent compelling. For most NDAs today, the manufacturer has outsourced much of the application, including the RCT itself. The application process has spawned a multibillion-dollar industry of companies that contract to perform the RCT, analyze the data, and assist the pharmaceutical firm in preparing and defending the NDA.

There are many CROs, some of which are somehow integrated into academic health centers. I have had, and voiced, concerns about this arrangement from the start, and I was there at the start. The patriarch of the CRO industry was Dennis Gillings, who was junior faculty with me, a colleague who collaborated on research projects and a book before his consulting to the pharmaceutical industry grew into Quintiles Transnational, Inc. My qualms about the marriage between pharmaceutical firms and CROs relate to conflicts of interest. So much has been written about this issue that I need not decry the fashion in which the pharmaceutical industry's business model is driven by profits and profit margins. The CRO functions in the service of that business model.

Science tests null hypotheses: a negative result is assumed and a positive result is a surprise. The business model wants and expects a positive result and is disappointed when none is forthcoming; often this is a very costly disappointment. One might well imagine that the corporate responses of the manufacturer and the CRO to a positive result would be more conducive to negotiating another contract than they would be to a negative result. A negative result might make a competing CRO seem more appealing. Given the judgment involved in analyzing the enormous data sets generated by large RCTs, one need not postulate malfeasance to imagine some prejudice at work. There is no mystery that whenever one compares RCTs supported by industry with RCTs supported by public moneys for the same drug, the same class of drug, or even the meta-analyses on the same class of drug, the industry-supported studies are more likely to be positive. I have illustrated this with much more than the literature on regional backache in *Worried Sick*.[32]

We are institutionalizing conflicts of interest. It starts with the fashion in which RCTs are outsourced and percolates down to the academic health centers,[33] on through the "thought leaders" to the practicing doctors. I countenance none of it.[34] We can do much if we tackle the fountainhead. We will go a long way just by demanding effectiveness trials. It is much harder to torture data to produce a large effect than to produce a small effect, and I don't value the latter.

In keeping with the contemporary communitarian ethic, it makes sense to me that pharmaceutical firms are in the private sector. Licensing their products, however, is a public-sector function, and I argue that modern RCTs are also a public-sector responsibility. I suggest the establishment of clinimetrics centers at medical schools and national RCT steering committees. All these entities should be staffed by academicians committed to the relevant issues in epidemiology. There is no shortage of willing and competent academics. Furthermore, the effort might indeed prove far more academic to serve effectiveness than to serve profitability. Funding for the staffing should be from federal coffers; the cost will be more than compensated by the savings that derive from keeping ineffective and me-too drugs from the nation's medicine chests. The steering committees would prioritize RCTs by promise and need and offer the clinimetrics centers the opportunity to bid to participate. The clinimetrics centers would function as public CROs and as the only agent to prepare and submit the NDAs. When we were in our youth, well before he founded Quintiles, Dennis Gillings and I formulated a very efficient RCT design that called for treating each of a small number of centers, each with a small number of subjects, as individual data points.[35] Such a design speaks to generalizability of results while rendering the process much more efficient than what is going on today.

The Insurance Industry and the Many Moral Hazards

The insurance industry is its own fortress, but we must confront it. There is a general belief that health-insurance companies have our interests at heart and place them at the forefront of their business models. That was my assumption, too, when I decided to analyze the U.S. "health-care system" for myself a decade ago. I had been invited to speak before congressional committees, the Social Security Advisory Board and other federal agencies, the National Business Group on Health, and various Conference Board and National League of Cities meetings. Several Fortune 50 executives responsible for benefits programs took me under their wings. And then I was invited to spend time with many of the leaders of the health-insurance industry, such as William McGuire (then of United Healthcare), members of the Consortium Health Group (the Blues), Cigna executives and their large clients, and more. Today, no vestige of naiveté remains. The needs, wants, and expectations of the clients, claimants, and beneficiaries are barely discernible and certainly not a high priority in today's corporate models and corporate ethics. We are being bamboozled.

The majority of the people in the United States who have health or workers' compensation insurance are insured by their employer and serviced by their insurance company. A minority are self-insured and serviced by their insurance company. If I need a heart transplantation, Blue Cross and Blue Shield of North Carolina passes the $500,000 cost on to my employer, the state of North Carolina, as an addition to the premium. The insurance company negotiates a fee, some percentage of the total cost, and takes that off the top of the money that flows from the employer to the providers. If I were self-employed and had purchased my own policy, the pool of the self-insured would be expected to cover the additional expense of the heart transplant. That is why my policy costs the state some $6,000 per year, whereas it would cost three to four times that amount if I were to purchase it on my own. But that's the least of the nefarious features.

The predominance of the former arrangement, in which the employer is essentially self-insured, creates a conflict for the insurer. As more money is spent on "health care," more flows into the coffers of the insurer to pay the enormous salaries and other aspects of "overhead" that are features of this industry, whether the entity is legally profit making or nominally "not-for-profit." Why do you think the health-insurance companies are so willing to promote screening programs and to underwrite the most expensive of me-too agents and unproved devices and procedures? Nearly all screening, from cholesterol to PSA (prostate-specific antigen) to mammography, leads to marginal benefit, if any, for the screened but to much largesse for the screeners and even more for the underwriters.

The Centers for Medicare and Medicaid Services (CMS), the federal agency that administers Medicare, is faced with enormous political pressures as to what should be covered and at what cost. A single-payer insurance system is long overdue. At issue is who decides what is to be paid for and how much to pay. Imagine the escalation in the activities of lobbyists and political action committees if the single payer was a federal agency. And the HMOs are not spared either. Executives from Kaiser on the West Coast once flew into Chapel Hill to discuss the rational management of back pain and some other issues. I asked them why they offered something like PSA screening given they were fully up to speed on its severe limitations as a screening test and its consequences for their membership, let alone their budgets. The answer was that competing health-care systems in their localities would accuse them of rationing care otherwise and would gain a competitive advantage.

Then there is the most egregious of the insurance models: the model for workers' compensation. Again, the majority of the expense is taken on by the large employers who insure the larger workforces. Again, the insurance company profits the more claims are processed. However, this industry has an actuarial model for disability insurance. The business model demands that all funds be collected at the outset to cover the pension for the duration of any long-term disability. These firms have war chests that we tend to learn about in economic downturns when their investments sour. As long as industry can pay the premiums, there is no financial disincentive for workers' compensation insurers to truly reform the contest of maximum medical improvement or the vortex of disability determination that we discussed earlier. They are cash cows for the workers' compensation insurance industry.

The rationale for insurance is that we share the risks of the catastrophes that might befall and decimate any one of us. In the early days of the insurance industry, there were fears that someone who needed money would torch his or her house, the so-called moral-hazard argument. The moral-hazard concept pertained to the claimant. That is not how I see it. The moral hazard pertains much more to the other stakeholders to varying degrees. Kafka understood this.

Much has been written about disparities in health care, usually focusing on issues in access or lack thereof. We have examined another disparity: if you're a workers' compensation claimant with a regional back "injury" in the contest of maximum medical improvement, you are entitled to everything available to heal your injury. Furthermore, refusing treatment is not an option that is applauded as evidence of good judgment; it's evidence of noncompliance. The result is far more iatrogenicity than the iatrogenicity for which all others with regional back pain are at risk. It makes no sense to stratify entitlement to the best money can buy. A rational health-care system entitles everyone to effectiveness and value.

We have already examined the rationale for basing disability determination on the quantification of impairment. No rationale exists. Basing the decision that someone is disabled on the magnitude of discernible disease (damage) is simply invalid. It belongs in the archives, and the industry it supports deserves to be a historical footnote. There is a better way.

And finally, a word about tort insurance. Much is known of the illness experience and much is known about redress for personal injury; it is clear that these two stations in life are simply incompatible. The former calls for coping skills, while the latter elicits symptom magnification. Symptom alleviation in the former is a triumph; in the latter it is costly. No-fault schemes are a better way.

Health Assurance and Disease Insurance

I have been honing an approach to rational reform of the health-care system based on the above considerations for some time. The effort takes advantage of insights gained from firsthand analysis of the sociopolitical constraints placed on clinical judgment and patient care by the workers' compensation systems of eight other countries. It takes into account an analysis of medicalization and Type II Medical Malpractice put forth in my earlier books, and it takes into account all that has been put forth in this book.

Most models for reform are not viable because of fiscal and political constraints. I have presented earlier versions to a number of leading scholars and several state agencies. And I have published an earlier iteration that was designed to be a private-sector alternative and to be offered to the uninsured workforce.[36] I have neither heard nor can I conjure up a substantive criticism to this approach, but I was not surprised when pressures were brought to squelch it even in the one state in which legislation tolerates innovation for the uninsured workforce. I am fully aware that this is not a fine-tuning or a tweaking but a thoroughgoing change that will dramatically affect the incomes and lifestyles of almost everyone gainfully involved in the status quo. Very few will come out better financially. However, all will find their roles clarified in an institution that serves the communitarian ethic by putting the health and welfare of the citizenry first. All will earn gratitude and respect by participating in a service profession that truly serves. The pride in and pleasure from this work that have eroded in the past fifty years will return. I may not live long enough to see it through to fulfillment, but I can hope to see it stir.

Given the experience with private-sector reform, I propose a state-based system for assuring health and insuring disease. The less-populous states may need to cooperate to reach a critical mass of more than 10 million people, but it is important that the national system operate as a conglomerate of independent units. This has nothing to do with market considerations; I have no need to demonstrate yet again that free-market principles do not apply to health care in the United States. Rather, the multiplication in the system is to serve the range of philosophies of well-being that this reform countenances.

Each state will create an enablement fund. It may be more palatable, given the precedents, if this fund is a percentage of wages (12 percent), but a comparable fund can derive from income taxation. By comparison, this is far less than what we currently expend on "health insurance." The moneys will distribute to two accounts: a disease-insurance account and a health-assurance account. The disease-insurance account is a shared risk pool designed to supplant health insurance as we know it for all citizens until one is eligible for federal Medicare insurance. The health-assurance account is not a shared risk pool. It is the repository for all moneys not expended from the disease-insurance account. Ownership in the health-assurance account is prorated to contributions. The health-assurance account is available for licensed services in the state relating to health and that are not underwritten by the disease-insurance account. This will become clear below.

The Disease-Insurance Account

The intellectual engine for managing the disease-insurance account is the same local clinimetrics center discussed above as participating in multi-site-effectiveness RCTs. The process must be as free of conflicts of interest as possible. There are two safeguards built into the system. One relates to the ability to compare administrative decisions across the states. The other follows from the clinimetrics center's fiduciary role. The size of the enablement fund is fixed by the gross domestic product of the state. The administration of the disease-insurance account cannot spend more than the fund has available. Furthermore, the administration cannot "save" money; money not expended in the disease-insurance account reverts to the health-assurance account. Nonetheless, there will be regulations that make accepting gifts, consultative fees, and the like illegal activities. Furthermore, the professional staff of the clinimetrics center will include dedicated full-time epidemiologists and statisticians, along with rotating full-time clinicians with epidemiology training and focus. As mentioned before, there is no manpower shortage.

The guiding principle of the disease-insurance account is to indemnify all that is demonstrated to be effective. The exercise is to calculate NNTs by taking advantage of evidence statements from the Cochrane Collaboration, the ACP Journal Club, the FDA's trial-data repository, and whatever else might be relevant without duplicating these available and ongoing evidence exercises. Agreeing on prerequisite NNTs for effectiveness requires a good deal of consensus building in each clinimetrics center.

1. As illustrated in the examples above, there is variability in the magnitude of effect between the trials that find evidence for an effect. Hence, there is often a range of NNTs.
2. What NNT does one need in order to declare the effectiveness clinically meaningful? I, and most others who are students of this exercise, would argue that an NNT of fifty is the upper limit of reliability and of meaningfulness. This means that a physician would need to treat fifty people for one of them to stand a good chance of benefiting. I would personally be more comfortable with an NNT of twenty or less for my cutoff. This is an issue in philosophy (and cost, as we'll discuss), but it is also an issue in the effect being measured. These cutoffs are defensible when the outcome is "hard"

(unequivocal), such as death, heart attack, end-stage renal disease, and the like. But here, too, there is a proviso: the effect has to be clinically meaningful in the context of life-course epidemiology. If the intervention spares one in twenty from death by colon cancer but spares none of these from death by something else at the same time (all-cause mortality), the clinically meaningful NNT is not twenty, since there is no meaningful result. Death is death.

3. NNTs for "soft" outcomes are more problematic. How much better do you have to make patients with rheumatoid arthritis feel, and how many patients must you treat, before you would consider the effectiveness clinically meaningful? That depends in part on the reliability and validity of the measure of subjective improvement. If there is a reasonable measure, how many more patients must improve when treated with an active agent rather than with a placebo or an old standby? Again, consensus must be reached as to the quality of these measures and their relevance to clinical effectiveness before analytic modeling is sensible.[37] That consensus will always be more severe than for "hard" outcomes; NNTs of five are likely.

4. The derivation and analysis of NNTs must be undertaken for a large but finite number of interventions and then must be repeated periodically as new data appear. I suspect a well-staffed clinimetrics center could handle a quarter of the clinical circumstances each year. Realize that most analyses find evidence lacking or absent, thereby rendering the effectiveness exercise perfunctory.

The clinimetrics center has two other functions relating to the disease-insurance account. First, a good deal of the practice of medicine that is "common practice" has never been subjected to scientific testing and may never be. Is such to be indemnified, and to what extent? Second, the center has to interact with the national RCT steering committee regarding participation in RCTs to test the effectiveness of new agents and devices.

A prime example of common practice is the clinical interview. The clinical interview is the essence of the medical treatment act. Someone has to listen to the "chief complaint," place that complaint into a clinical context, and act on the context. Most of the process can be subjected to scientific testing as to efficacy, efficiency, reliability, and even effectiveness. But not all can be studied. The clinical interview does much more than collect data relevant to the differential diagnosis; it establishes the trust that is necessary for medical decision making. True, medical decision making is simplified by expunging the ineffective from the menu that is indemnified. Some might argue that computerized decision aids are the answer, but I am a serious doubter and in good company.[38]

I suspect that "decision aids" will be useful only when the decision lends itself to the kind of analytic approach the clinimetrics center is taking to the issue of effectiveness. The clinimetrics center is a de facto decision aid. There is much more to the experience of illness, however, from semiotics to the making of decisions when the data are inadequate. That is when you need a physician. As Robert McNutt argues, for the patient to remain the pilot, there must be access to a caring, thoughtful, experienced navigator.[39] I would argue that everyone should have an hour of medical interview underwritten for each year of adult life. If you do not need a clinical interview until you are forty, you will have accumulated nineteen hours (or more, depending on the definition of adulthood) of clinical interview time to be used as needed. I mean "as needed" since, based on NNTs, there is no reason to underwrite a routine annual examination. If one is worried, though, that is a legitimate "need" and one that may be well served.[40]

Another prime example of common practice is not as common as it should be: psychological counseling. The saga of regional low back pain would not be as convoluted if some or all could find their way into productive counseling. No one has been able to design a trial that demonstrates effectiveness of such counseling, let alone cost-effectiveness, because of all the vagaries related to practice style, client differences, and outcome measures. As with the clinical interview, I am strongly prejudiced toward a belief in the value of "talk therapy" with someone who is prepared to be helpful. It is not expensive: for the salary of one overpaid hospital administrator, you could hire ten to twenty social workers, give each a case load of ten to twenty struggling families, and, even if only a minority of the families were helped, make a very important difference. And for one year of useless interventional cardiology and cardiovascular surgery at my hospital, we could employ great teams of social workers. Therefore, everyone insured under the disease-insurance account has an evaluative hour underwritten each year and short-term intervention when indicated.

The clinimetrics centers will be offered the opportunity to participate in RCTs that have been prioritized by the national RCT steering committees. Agreeing to be a participating center is a challenging and complex decision. The center will be recruiting patients from its catchment area, organizing data collection and analysis, and paying for patient care. The last is less of a burden for a pharmaceutical since the agent is supplied gratis from the manufacturer, but monitoring for effects can be expensive. For RCTs of devices and procedures, the underwriting can entail substantial sums for patient care. "Finder fees" and other inducements will be history once the ethics of this approach to medical progress are incorporated into the fabric of American life. So the clinimetrics center has to revisit the thinking of the national RCT steering committee. If the agent under study proves effective, will it be of enough value to enough people in the state account to justify participating in the trial, or are resources better spent participating in a different trial?

Speaking of money and resources, there is no doubt that there will be enormous savings when the enablement fund replaces the current mess. The bizarrely expensive business of NDAs will be streamlined. The marketing and "educational" budgets of manufacturers and providers will become transparent and easy to regulate. Nearly all elective high-ticket items will no longer be underwritten. Based on the analysis of the topics considered in *Worried Sick*, the per capita annual expenditure from the disease-insurance account today would not exceed $1,000 with the current pricing schedule.[41] Furthermore, starting this account from scratch allows for innovative and cost-saving Internet technologies that will eliminate a good deal of the current administrative overhead.

Furthermore, the disease-insurance account is in a position to be very proactive in regard to cost-effectiveness beyond excluding the ineffective. There is no reason to tolerate the repugnant incomes garnered by many employed by the "health-care" industry. The disease-insurance account can stipulate the overhead percentage it is willing to underwrite. Furthermore, it is straightforward to add cost to the NNT by applying the COPE (cost of preventing an event) statistic, which factors the cost of the treatment into the NNT.[42]

There is no reason why the account could not negotiate with purveyors based on the cost-effectiveness of the intervention. For example, TNF-alpha inhibitors are biotechnology triumphs that lead to important symptomatic improvement in about half of patients with active rheumatoid arthritis unresponsive to traditional agents. These are effective agents. They cost over $10,000 per year. Rheumatoid arthritis afflicts 1 percent of the population but is not a severe progressive disease in most. The agents are marvels, but the intellectual wherewithal to develop them derived from Nobel Prize– and Lasker Award–winning contributions from government-supported laboratories. There is no advantage to the disease-insurance account to underwrite the marketing budgets of the manufacturers, or their "educational budgets," or the outrageousness of their profit margin. An NNT-COPE calculation would justify a price that is a fraction of the current price, and the disease-insurance account should demand such in a very public fashion.

Notice that I am not recommending the notion of "co-pay." If the intervention is effective, it is provided. However, I fear as great a backlash from stakeholders in the current system, including all the providers and purveyors of the ineffective, a backlash that could prove litigious. My solution is to have two levels of co-pay: 0 percent or 100 percent. If the patient insists on something that is not covered and therefore requires 100 percent co-pay because it is deemed to offer inadequate effectiveness, he or she will be so informed—and informed as well that there is a fallback in the health-assurance account, as we will discuss. Notice, too, that I am not countenancing stratified health care. The disease-insurance account underwrites what is effective for patients whether they are employed, unemployed, injured, or disabled. What has been indemnified by Medicaid and workers' compensation along with all the flavors of private "health" indemnity will fall under the disease-insurance account. Ethical medical ministration knows no such distinctions.

The Health-Assurance Account

Health is difficult to define. I take comfort in the fact that even the late Hans-Georg Gadamer, a twentieth-century philosopher of great reputation, had difficulty understanding how physicians could stare into "the face of illness . . . to discover the great enigma of health." In 1991 he stated that "the fundamental fact remains that it is illness and not health which 'objectifies' itself, which confronts us as something opposed to us and which forces itself on us. . . . The real mystery lies in the hidden character of health."[43] Eighteen years later, health is still an enigma, but not the enigma it once was. Life-course epidemiology has unraveled some of the mystery, though not the underlying mechanisms. Health in the resource-advantaged world requires the wherewithal to feel comfortable in one's own skin. You need to find a station in your community that satisfies to an important degree. You need to be able to maintain that station by virtue of the earnings from work that satisfies you to an important degree. You need to have the personal resources to cope with the predicaments that are bound to come up. High on this list of predicaments are the occasional encounters with painful episodes, and regional low back pain is firmly and prominently entrenched among these. Health does not require low cholesterol, low blood pressure, low body-mass index, normal kidney function, normal cardiac output, or other physiological measurements. It is the erosion of these that is prerequisite to disease. You can have rheumatoid arthritis and still have your health if you are a *person* with rheumatoid arthritis and not a "rheumatoid."

The health-assurance account exists to foster your health. It accumulates based on your contribution to the enablement fund minus the expenditures of the disease-insurance account. It is managed like a state retirement fund. But it is yours on a prorated basis to use however you wish for health-related (as defined above) services that are provided by licensed professionals in your state. If you never touch it, it will revert to your pension at retirement. If you are not convinced that cholesterol screening or coronary artery stents are as ineffective as determined by the clinimetrics center, you can use your health-assurance account funds toward the purchase of them outside the disease-insurance account.

The health-assurance account will have an advisory component. If you are an entry-level employee, it might be very wise for you to expend health-assurance funds for instruction in English as a second language or to acquire skills that afford job mobility. These moneys are available to aid you if you don't otherwise have the wherewithal for attaining a station in life that promotes your healthfulness. There is also a role for the health-assurance account in educating the public as to the hazards of not attaining a satisfying station in life. It has proved possible to use such a campaign to change the social construction of regional back "injury" in other countries.[44] We need to consider how to generalize that educational experience to much more than back pain.

The Disabled, the Disallowed, the Disaffected, and the Disavowed

The determination of disability, which we discussed at length in chapters 7 and 8, has left many an insight in its turbulent wake. Specialized physician skills are not particularly relevant to disability determination. However, a caring society can mobilize a jury of peers that might be a match for the task. Many European countries rely on this mechanism, and so do we in the United States, since any appeal of a denial ends up in nonmedical adjudication—albeit often with confusing medical input. I do not think we the people would have much difficulty giving a pension under SSDI or SSI to someone we felt incapable of substantial gainful activity. We would need testimony, perhaps from the applicant or the relevant community, but we could try to listen to the narratives fully and hope to conclude wisely. We might be fooled and flummoxed, but I doubt this would be a frequent occurrence, and I am sure that going to great lengths in trying to establish veracity would do more harm to the process than catching the occasional thief would serve our communitarian ethic. As for the injured worker, a combination of a liberal "schedule" for overt damage and enforced safety regulation makes perfect sense. Predicaments of life such as back pain are not "injuries."

These are the easy issues. One lesson of this book is that many people claim disability awards because they are disaffected and have been disallowed access to a station in life where they might not feel so estranged. Impairment-based disability determination has turned medicine into the agent of the state in ways that make the claimant sicker. Medicine needs to refuse such a role and earn the trustworthiness to advise these patients and to explain their circumstances to society at large. The health-assurance account is designed to promote options other than a disability claim, which is often futile and nearly always a barrier to recovery. There should be other mechanisms to provide such a resource for those who have not earned ownership in the health-assurance account, some state fund that provides for them and subsidizes their membership in the disease-insurance account without the stigmatization and inadequate care that Medicaid currently underwrites.

It is a very long tunnel, but there is a light at the end.

NOTES

Abbreviations

Ann Intern Med	*Annals of Internal Medicine*
Ann Rheum Dis	*Annals of Rheumatic Diseases*
Arthritis Care Res	*Arthritis Care and Research*
Arthritis Rheum	*Arthritis and Rheumatism*
BMJ	*British Medical Journal*
JAMA	*Journal of the American Medical Association*
J Occup Environ Med	*Journal of Occupational and Environmental Medicine*
J Rheumatol	*Journal of Rheumatology*
N Engl J Med	*New England Journal of Medicine*
Occup Environ Med	*Occupational and Environmental Medicine*

Introduction

1   N. M. Hadler, "Regional Back Pain," *N Engl J Med* 315 (1986): 1090–92.

2   N. M. Hadler, R. C. Tait, and J. T. Chibnall, "Back Pain in the Workplace," *JAMA* 297 (2007): 1594–96; N. M. Hadler, *Occupational Musculoskeletal Disorders*, 3rd ed. (Philadelphia: Lippincott Williams & Wilkins, 2005).

3   N. M. Hadler, "A Ripe Old Age," *Archives of Internal Medicine* 163 (2003): 1261–62; N. M. Hadler, *The Last Well Person: How to Stay Well Despite the Health-Care System* (Montreal: McGill-Queens University Press, 2004).

4   N. M. Hadler, *Worried Sick: A Prescription for Health in an Overtreated America* (Chapel Hill: University of North Carolina Press, 2008).

Chapter One

1   P. W. Brandt-Rauf and S. I. Brandt-Rauf, "History of Occupational Medicine: Relevance of Imhotep and the Edwin Smith Papyrus," *British Journal of Industrial Medicine* 44 (1987): 68–70.

2 O. Sugar, "Charles Lasègue and His 'Considerations on Sciatica,'" *JAMA* 253 (1985): 1767–68.

3 T. Keller and T. Chappell, "The Rise and Fall of Erichsen's Disease (Railroad Spine)," *Spine* 21 (1996): 1597–1601.

4 E. Caplan, "Trains, Brains, and Sprains: Railway Spine and the Origins of Psychoneuroses," *Bulletin of the History of Medicine* 69 (1995): 387–420.

5 T. McCrae, *Sir William Osler's "The Principles and Practice of Medicine,"* 10th ed. (New York: Appleton, 1926), pp. 1141–44.

6 H. Beck, *The Origins of the Authoritarian Welfare State in Prussia* (Ann Arbor: University of Michigan Press, 1995), p. 120.

7 W. J. Mixter and J. S. Barr, "Rupture of the Intervertebral Disc with Involvement of the Spinal Canal," *N Engl J Med* 211 (1934): 210–15.

8 T. Brown, J. C. Nemiah, and J. S. Barr, "Psychologic Factors in Low-Back Pain," *N Engl J Med* 251 (1954): 123–28.

Chapter Two

1 L. M. Verbrugge and F. J. Ascione, "Exploring the Iceberg: Common Symptoms and How People Care for Them," *Medical Care* 25 (1987): 539–69.

2 T. W. Strine and J. M. Hootman, "U.S. National Prevalence and Correlates of Low Back and Neck Pain among Adults," *Arthritis Rheum (Arthritis Care Res)* 57 (2007): 656–65.

3 K. T. Palmer, K. Walsh, H. Bendall, C. Cooper, and D. Coggon, "Back Pain in Britain: Comparison of Two Prevalence Surveys at an Interval of 10 Years," *BMJ* 320 (2000): 1577–78.

4 P. Croft, "Is Life Becoming More of a Pain?," *BMJ* 320 (2000): 1552–53.

5 H. Raspe, C. Matthis, P. Croft, T. O'Neill, and the European Vertebral Osteoporosis Study Group, "Variation in Back Pain between Countries: The Example of Britain and Germany," *Spine* 29 (2004): 1017–21.

6 Ibid.

Chapter Three

1 J. D. Cassidy, P. Côté, L. J. Carroll, and V. Kristman, "Incidence and Course of Low Back Pain Episodes in the General Population," *Spine* 30 (2005): 2817–23.

2 J. A. Kopec, E. C. Sayre, and J. M. Esdaile, "Predictors of Back Pain in a General Population Cohort," *Spine* 29 (2004): 70–78.

3 T. S. Carey, A. Evans, N. Hadler, W. Kalsbeek, C. McLaughlin, and J. Fryer, "Care-Seeking among Individuals with Chronic Low Back Pain," *Spine* 20 (1995): 312–17.

4 D. Carnes, S. Parsons, D. Ashby, A. Breen, N. E. Foster, T. Pincus, S. Vogel, and M. Underwood, "Chronic Musculoskeletal Pain Rarely Presents in a Single Body Site: Results for the UK Population Study," *Rheumatology* 46 (2007): 1168–70.

5 I. Hacking, *The Social Construction of What?* (Cambridge, Mass.: Harvard University Press, 2000).

6 M. Foucault, *The Birth of the Clinic: An Archaeology of Medical Perception* (New York: Vintage Books, 1973).

7 E. Freidson, *Medical Work in America: Essays on Health Care* (New Haven: Yale University Press, 1989).

8 P. Starr, *The Social Transformation of American Medicine* (New York: Basic Books, 1982).

9 K. K. Barker, *The Fibromyalgia Story: Medical Authority and Women's Worlds of Pain* (Philadelphia: Temple University Press, 2005).

10 D. Mechanic, "Response Factors in Illness: The Study of Illness Behavior," *Social Psychiatry and Psychiatric Epidemiology* 1 (1966): 11–20.

11 N. M. Hadler and G. E. Ehrlich, "Fibromyalgia and the Conundrum of Disability Determination," *J Occup Environ Med* 45 (2003): 1030–33.

12 N. M. Hadler, "If You Have to Prove You Are Ill, You Can't Get Well: The Object Lesson of 'Fibromyalgia,'" *Spine* 21 (1996): 2396–400.

13 C. R. Chapman and J. Gavrin, "Suffering: The Contributions of Persistent Pain," *Lancet* 353 (1999): 2233–37; E. J. Cassell, *The Nature of Suffering and the Goals of Medicine*, 2nd ed. (Oxford: Oxford University Press, 2004).

14 P. van Wilgen, M. W. van Ittersum, A. A. Kaptein, and M. van Wijhe, "Illness Perceptions in Patients with Fibromyalgia and Their Relationship to Quality of Life and Catastrophizing," *Arthritis Rheum* 58 (2008): 3618–26.

15 R. M. Kaplan, S. M. Schmidt, and T. A. Cronan, "Quality of Well Being in Patients with Fibromyalgia," *J Rheumatol* 27 (2000): 785–89.

16 F. Wolfe, H. A. Smythe, M. B. Yunus, and others, "The American College of Rheumatology 1990 Criteria for the Classification of Fibromyalgia," *Arthritis Rheum* 33 (1990): 160–72.

17 F. Wolfe, "Stop Using the American College of Rheumatology Criteria in the Clinic," *J Rheumatol* 30 (2003): 1671–72.

18 S. Bergman, P. Herrström, K. Högström, I. F. Petersson, B. Svensson, and L. T. H. Jacobsson, "Chronic Musculoskeletal Pain, Prevalence Rates, and Sociodemographic Associations in a Swedish Population Study," *J Rheumatol* 28 (2001): 1369–77; T. Schochat and C. Beckmann, "Sociodemographic Characteristics, Risk Factors, and Reproductive History in Subjects with Fibromyalgia: Results of a Population-Based Case-Control Study," *Zeitschrift für Rheumatologie* 62 (2003): 46–59.

19 K. P. White, W. R. Nielson, M. Harth, T. Ostbye, and M. Speechley, "Chronic Widespread Musculoskeletal Pain with or without Fibromyalgia: Psychological Distress in a Representative Community Adult Sample," *J Rheumatol* 29 (2002): 588–94.

20 I. M. Hunt, A. J. Silman, S. Benjamin, J. McBeth, and G. J. Macfarlane, "The Prevalence and Associated Features of Chronic Widespread Pain in the Community Using the 'Manchester' Definition of Chronic Widespread Pain," *Rheumatology* 38 (1998): 275–79.

21 G. E. Simon, M. VonKorff, M. Piccinelli, C. Fullerton, and J. Ormel, "An International Study of the Relation between Somatic Symptoms and Depression," *N Engl*

J Med 341 (1999): 1329–35; H. M. Nordahl and T. C. Stiles, "Personality Styles in Patients with Fibromyalgia, Major Depression, and Healthy Controls," *Annals of General Psychiatry* 6 (2007): 9 (DOI: 10.1186/1744-859X-6-9).

22 S. Benjamin, S. Morris, J. McBeth, G. J. Macfarlane, and A. J. Silman, "The Association between Chronic Widespread Pain and Mental Disorder," *Arthritis Rheum* 43 (2000): 561–67; K. G. Raphael, M. N. Janal, S. Nayak, J. E. Schwartz, and R. M. Gallagher, "Familial Aggregation of Depression in Fibromyalgia: A Community-Based Test of Alternative Hypotheses," *Pain* 110 (2004): 449–60.

23 A. L. Hassett, L. E. Simonelli, D. C. Radvanski, S. Buyske, S. V. Savage, and L. H. Sigal, "The Relationship between Affect Balance Style and Clinical Outcomes in Fibromyalgia," *Arthritis Rheum (Arthritis Care Res)* 59 (2008): 833–40.

24 S. Bergman, P. Herrström, L. T. H. Jacobsson, and I. F. Petersson, "Chronic Widespread Pain: A Three Year Follow-up of Pain Distribution and Risk Factors," *J Rheumatol* 29 (2002): 818–25; A. Kassam and S. B. Patten, "Major Depression, Fibromyalgia, and Labour Force Participation: A Population-Based Cross-Sectional Study," *BioMed Central Musculoskeletal Disorders* 7 (2006): 4 (DOI: 10.1186/1471-2474-7-4); M.-A. Fitzcharles, D. DaCosta, and R. Pöyhiä, "A Study of Standard Care in Fibromyalgia Syndrome: A Favorable Outcome," *J Rheumatol* 30 (2003): 154–59.

25 A. C. Papageorgiou, A. J. Silman, and G. J. Macfarlane, "Chronic Widespread Pain in the Population: A Seven Year Follow-up Study," *Ann Rheum Dis* 61 (2002): 1071–74.

26 G. J. Macfarlane, E. Thomas, A. C. Papageorgiou, J. Schollum, P. R. Croft, and A. J. Silman, "The Natural History of Chronic Pain in the Community: A Better Prognosis than in the Clinic?," *J Rheumatol* 23 (1996): 1617–20.

27 B. C. Kersh, L. A. Bradley, G. S. Alarcón, and others, "Psychosocial and Health Status Variables Independently Predict Health Care Seeking in Fibromyalgia," *Arthritis Care Res* 45 (2001): 362–711.

28 E. Scarry, *The Body in Pain: The Making and Unmaking of the World* (Oxford: Oxford University Press, 1985).

29 G. M. Aronoff, J. B. Feldman, and T. S. Campion, "Management of Chronic Pain and Control of Long-Term Disability," *Occupational Medicine* 15 (2000): 755–70.

30 R. R. Ferrari and A. S. Russell, "Fibromyalgia: 30 Years of Drug-Seeking Behavior," *Nature Clinical Practice Rheumatology* 3 (2007): 62–63.

31 R. Rey, *The History of Pain* (Cambridge: Harvard University Press, 1995).

32 A. J. Barsky, "The Patient with Hypochondriasis," *N Engl J Med* 345 (2001): 1395–99.

33 A. J. Barsky and J. F. Borus, "Functional Somatic Syndromes," *Ann Intern Med* 130 (1999): 910–21.

34 C. E. Rosenberg and J. Golden, eds., *Framing Disease: Studies in Cultural History* (New Brunswick: Rutgers University Press, 1992).

35 J. Stone, W. Wojcik, D. Durrance, and others, "What Should We Say to Patients with Symptoms Unexplained by Disease? The 'Number Needed to Offend,'" *BMJ* 325 (2002): 1449–50.

36 P. Watkins, "Medically Unexplained Symptoms," *Clinical Medicine (JRCPL)* 2 (2002): 389–90.

37 I. Hazemaijer and J. J. Rasker, "Fibromyalgia and the Therapeutic Domain: A Philosophical Study on the Origins of Fibromyalgia in a Specific Social Setting," *Rheumatology* 42 (2003): 507–15.

38 D. Mechanic, "Social Psychologic Factors Affecting the Presentation of Bodily Complaints," *N Engl J Med* 286 (1972): 1132–39.

39 D. J. Wallace and D. J. Clauw, eds., *Fibromyalgia and Other Central Pain Syndromes* (Philadelphia: Lippincott Williams & Wilkins, 2005).

40 N. M. Hadler, "Mongering Diseases to Hawk Pills: The Case of Fibromyalgia," *Public Citizen Health Research Group Health Letter* 24 (2008): 9–12.

41 N. M. Hadler and S. Greenhalgh, "Labeling Woefulness: The Social Construction of Fibromyalgia," *Spine* 30 (2005): 1–4.

42 S. Greenhalgh, *Under the Medical Gaze: Facts and Fictions of Chronic Pain* (Berkeley: University of California Press, 2001).

43 J. McBeth, D. P. Symmons, A. J. Silman, T. Allison, R. Webb, T. Brammah, and G. J. Macfarlane, "Musculoskeletal Pain Is Associated with Long-Term Increased Risk of Cancer and Cardiovascular-Related Mortality," *Rheumatology* 48 (2009): 74–77.

44 G. T. Jones, A. J. Silman, C. Power, and G. J. Macfarlane, "Are Common Symptoms in Childhood Associated with Chronic Widespread Body Pain in Adulthood?," *Arthritis Rheum* 56 (2007): 1669–75.

Chapter Four

1 R. A. Deyo, S. K. Mirza, and B. I. Martin, "Back Pain Prevalence and Visit Rates: Estimates from U.S. National Surveys, 2002," *Spine* 31 (2006): 2724–27.

2 J. Horal, "The Clinical Appearance of Low Back Disorders in the City of Gothenburg, Sweden: Comparisons of Incapacitated Probands with Matched Controls," *Acta Orthopaedica Scandinavica* 118, suppl. (1969): 1–109.

3 J. Smedley, H. Inskip, P. Buckle, C. Cooper, and D. Coggon, "Epidemiological Differences between Back Pain of Sudden and Gradual Onset," *J Rheumatol* 32 (2005): 528–32.

4 J. J. Liszka-Hackzell and D. P. Martin, "An Analysis of the Relationship between Activity and Pain in Chronic and Acute Low Back Pain," *Anesthesia and Analgesia* 9 (2004): 477–81.

5 E. M. Hagen, E. Svensen, H. R. Eriksen, C. M. Ihlebæk, and H. Ursin, "Comorbid Subjective Health Complaints in Low Back Pain," *Spine* 31 (2006): 1491–95.

6 H. M. Hadler, "Four Laws of Therapeutic Dynamics," *Journal of Occupational and Environmental Medicine* 39 (1997): 295–98.

7 B. W. Koes, M. W. van Tulder, R. Ostelo, A. K. Burton, and G. Waddell, "Clinical Guidelines for the Management of Low Back Pain in Primary Care: An International Comparison," *Spine* 26 (2001): 2504–14.

8 D. G. Borenstein, J. W. O'Mara, S. D. Boden, and others, "The Value of Magnetic Resonance Imaging of the Lumbar Spine to Predict Low-Back Pain in Asymptomatic Subjects," *Journal of Bone and Joint Surgery* (American) 83A (2001): 1306–11.

9 T. Videman, M. C. Battié, L. E. Gibbons, K. Maravilla, H. Manninen, and J. Kaprio,

"Associations between Back Pain History and Lumbar MRI Findings," *Spine* 28 (2003): 583–88.

10 J. G. Jarvik and R. A. Deyo, "Diagnostic Evaluation of Low Back Pain with Emphasis on Imaging," *Ann Intern Med* 137 (2002): 586–97.

11 P. Miller, D. Kendrick, E. Bentley, and K. Fielding, "Cost-effectiveness of Lumbar Spine Radiography in Primary Care Patients with Low Back Pain," *Spine* 27 (2002): 2391–97.

12 D. Kendrick, K. Fielding, E. Bentley, and others, "Radiography of the Lumbar Spine in Primary Care Patients with Low Back Pain: Randomized Controlled Trial," *BMJ* 322 (2001): 400–405.

13 J. D. Lurie, N. J. Birkmeyer, and J. N. Weinstein, "Rates of Advanced Spinal Imaging and Spine Surgery," *Spine* 28 (2003): 616–20.

14 T. S. Carey, M. Garrett, A. Jackman, and N. M. Hadler, "Recurrence and Care Seeking after Acute Back Pain," *Medical Care* 37 (1999): 157–64.

15 V. Sundararajn, T. R. Konrad, J. Garrett, and T. Carey, "Patterns and Determinants of Multiple Provider Use in Patients with Acute Low Back Pain," *Journal of General Internal Medicine* 13 (1998): 528–33.

16 L. Goubert, G. Crombez, and I. De Bourdeaudhuij, "Low Back Pain, Disability, and Back Pain Myths in a Community Sample: Prevalence and Interrelationships," *European Journal of Pain* 8 (2004): 385–94.

17 M. C. Battié and T. Videman, "Lumbar Disc Degeneration: Epidemiology and Genetics," *Journal of Bone and Joint Surgery* (American) 88 (2006): 3–9; M. C. Battié, T. Videman, J. Kaprio, and others, "The Twin Spine Study: Contributions to a Changing View of Disc Degeneration," *Spine Journal* 9 (2009): 47–59.

18 A. Levin, "The Cochrane Collaboration," *Ann Intern Med* 135 (2001): 309–12.

19 S. Mallett and M. Clarke, "How Many Cochrane Reviews Are Needed to Cover Existing Evidence on the Effects of Health Care Interventions?," ACP *Journal Club* 139 (2003): A-11–12.

20 G. H. Swingler, J. Volmink, and J. P. A. Ioannidis, "Number of Published Systematic Reviews and Global Burden of Disease: Database Analysis," *BMJ* 327 (2003): 1083–84.

21 L. M. Bouter, V. Pennick, and C. Bombardier, "Cochrane Back Review Group," *Spine* 28 (2003): 1215–18.

22 M. van Tulder, A. Furlan, C. Bombardier, and L. Bouter, "Updated Method Guidelines for Systematic Reviews in the Cochrane Collaboration Back Review Group," *Spine* 28 (2003): 1290–99.

23 P. H. Ferreira, M. L. Ferreira, C. G. Maher, K. Refshauge, R. D. Herbert, and J. Latimer, "Effect of Applying Different 'Levels of Evidence' Criteria on Conclusions of Cochrane Reviews of Interventions for Low Back Pain," *Journal of Clinical Epidemiology* 55 (2002): 1126–29.

24 L. P. Moja, E. Telaro, R. D'Amico, I. Moschetti, L. Coe, and A. Liberati, "Assessment of Methodological Quality of Primary Studies by Systematic Reviews: Results of the Metaquality Cross-Sectional Study," *BMJ* 330 (2005): 1053–55.

25 A. Jørgensen, J. Hilden, and P. Gøtzsche, "Cochrane Reviews Compared with

Industry Supported Meta-Analyses and Other Meta-Analyses of the Same Drugs: Systematic Review," *BMJ* 332 (2006): 782–86.

26 M. W. van Tulder, T. Touray, A. D. Furlan, S. Solway, and L. M. Bouter, "Muscle Relaxants for Non-specific Low Back Pain," Cochrane Database of Systematic Reviews (2003), issue 4, art. no. CD004252, DOI: 10.1002/14651858.CD004252.

27 T. Sahar, M. J. Cohen, V. Ne'eman, L. Kandel, D. O. Odebiyi, I. Lev, M. Brezis, and A. Lahad, "Insoles for Prevention and Treatment of Back Pain," Cochrane Database of Systematic Reviews (2007), issue 4, art. no. CD005275, DOI: 10.1002/14651858. CD005275.pub2.

28 J. A. Clarke, M. W. van Tulder, S. E. I. Blomberg, H. C. W. de Vet, G. J. M. G. van der Heijden, G. Bronfort, and L. M. Bouter, "Traction for Low-Back Pain with or without Sciatica," Cochrane Database of Systematic Reviews (2007), issue 2, art. no. CD003010, DOI: 10.1002/14651858.CD003010.pub4.

29 S. D. French, M. Cameron, B. F. Walker, J. W. Reggars, and A. J. Esterman, "Superficial Heat or Cold for Low Back Pain," Cochrane Database of Systematic Reviews (2006), issue 1, art. no. CD004750, DOI: 10.1002/14651858.CD004750.pub2.

30 J. Gabbay and A. le May, "Evidence-Based Guidelines or Collectively Constructed 'Mindlines'? Ethnographic Study of Knowledge Management in Primary Care," *BMJ* 329 (2004): 1013–16.

31 Quebec Task Force of Spinal Disorders, "Scientific Approach to the Assessment and Management of Activity-Related Spinal Disorders," *Spine* 12, suppl. 1 (1987): S1–59.

32 S. Bigos, O. Bowyer, G. Braen, and others, "Acute Low Back Problems in Adults," Clinical Practice Guideline no. 14, AHCPR Publication no. 95–0642 (Rockville, Md.: Agency for Health Care Policy and Research, Public Health Service, U.S. Department of Health and Human Services, December 1994).

33 E. G. Gonzalez and R. S. Materson, eds., *The Nonsurgical Management of Acute Low Back Pain: Cutting through the* AHCPR *Guidelines* (New York: Demos, 1997).

34 N. Freemantle, "Commentary: Is NICE Delivering the Goods?," *BMJ* 329 (2004): 1003–4.

35 R. Taylor and J. Giles, "Cash Interests Taint Drug Advice," *Nature* 437 (2005): 1070–71.

36 R. Chou, A. Qaseem, V. Snow, and others, "Diagnosis and Treatment of Low Back Pain: A Joint Clinical Practice Guideline for the American College of Physicians and the American Pain Society," *Ann Intern Med* 147 (2007): 478–91; R. Chou and L. H. Huffman, "Nonpharmacologic Therapies for Acute and Chronic Low Back Pain: A Review of the Evidence for an American Pain Society/American College of Physicians Clinical Practice Guideline," *Ann Intern Med* 147 (2007): 492–504; R. Chou and L. H. Huffman, "Medications for Acute and Chronic Low Back Pain: A Review of the Evidence for an American Pain Society/American College of Physicians Clinical Practice Guideline," *Ann Intern Med* 147 (2007): 505–14.

37 S. J. Linton, "A Review of Psychological Risk Factors in Back and Neck Pain," *Spine* 25 (2000): 1148–56; M. A. Adams, A. F. Mannion, and P. Dolan, "Personal Risk Factors for First-Time Low Back Pain," *Spine* 24 (1999): 2497–505.

38 W. E. Hoogendoorn, M. N. M. van Poppel, P. M. Bongers, B. W. Koes, and L. M. Bouter, "Systematic Review of Psychosocial Factors at Work and Private Life as Risk Factors for Back Pain," *Spine* 25 (2000): 2114–25.

39 P. R. Croft, A. C. Papagerogiou, S. Ferry, E. Thomas, M. I. V. Jayson, and J. F. Silman, "Psychological Distress and Low Back Pain: Evidence from a Prospective Cohort Study in the General Population," *Spine* 20 (1995): 2731–37.

40 T. Pincus, A. K. Burton, S. Vogel, and A. P. Field, "A Systematic Review of Psychological Factors as Predictors of Chronicity/Disability in Prospective Cohorts of Low Back Pain," *Spine* 27 (2002): E109–20.

41 N. M. Hadler, "Rheumatology and the Health of the Workforce," *Arthritis Rheum* 44 (2001): 1971–74.

42 N. M. Hadler, "The Injured Worker and the Internist," *Ann Intern Med* 120 (1994): 163–64.

43 M. von Korff, W. Barlow, D. Cherkin, and R. Deyo, "Effects of Practice Style in Managing Back Pain," *Ann Intern Med* 121 (1994): 187–95.

44 M. von Korff, J. E. Moore, K. Lorig, and others, "A Randomized Trial of a Lay Person–Led Self-Management Group Intervention for Back Pain Patients in Primary Care," *Spine* 23 (1998): 2608–15.

45 C. J. Main and A. C. Williams, "Musculoskeletal Pain," *BMJ* 325 (2002): 534–37; C. J. Main, "Early Psychosocial Interventions for Low Back Pain in Primary Care," *BMJ* 331 (2005): 88.

46 P. Jellema, D. A. W. M. van der Windt, H. E. van der Horst, J. W. R. Twisk, W. A. B. Stalman, and L. M. Bouter, "Should Treatment of (Sub)acute Low Back Pain Be Aimed at Psychosocial Prognostic Factors? Cluster Randomised Clinical Trial in General Practice," *BMJ* 331 (2005): 84–87.

47 D. van der Windt, E. Hay, P. Jellema, and C. Main, "Psychosocial Interventions for Low Back Pain in Primary Care," *Spine* 33 (2008): 81–89.

Chapter Five

1 R. Ferrari, A. S. Russell, L. J. Carroll, and J. D. Cassidy, "A Reexamination of the Whiplash Associated Disorders (WAD) as a Systemic Illness," *Ann Rheum Dis* 64 (2005): 1337–42.

2 A. Malleson, *Whiplash and Other Useful Illnesses* (Montreal: McGill-Queen's University Press, 2002).

3 M. Partheni, C. Constantoyannis, R. Ferrari, and others, "A Prospective Cohort Study of the Outcome of Acute Whiplash Injury in Greece," *Clinical and Experimental Rheumatology* 18 (2000): 67–70.

4 R. Ferrari and C. Lang, "A Cross-Cultural Comparison between Canada and Germany of Symptom Expectation for Whiplash Injury," *Journal of Spinal Disorders and Techniques* 18 (2005): 92–97.

5 A. Russell and R. Ferrari, "Whiplash: Social Interventions and Solutions," *J Rheumatol* 35 (2008): 2300–302.

6 A. A. Berglund, L. Alfredsson, J. D. Cassidy, and others, "The Association between

Exposure to a Rear-End Collision and Future Neck or Shoulder Pain: A Cohort Study," *Journal of Clinical Epidemiology* 53 (2000): 1089–94.

7 J. D. Cassidy, L. Carroll, P. Cote, and others, "Effect of Eliminating Compensation for Pain and Suffering on the Outcome of Insurance Claims for Whiplash Injury," *N Engl J Med* 342 (2000): 1179–86.

8 A. Berglund, L. Alfredsson, I. Jensen, J. D. Cassidy, and Å. Nygren, "The Association between Exposure to a Rear-End Collision and Future Health Complaints," *Journal of Clinical Epidemiology* 54 (2001): 851–56.

9 J. D. Cassidy, L. Carroll, P. Côté, A. Berglund, and Å Nygren, "Low Back Pain after Traffic Collisions: A Population-Based Cohort Study," *Spine* 28 (2003): 1002–9.

10 L. H. Pobereskin, "Whiplash following Rear End Collisions: A Prospective Cohort Study," *Journal of Neurology, Neurosurgery, and Psychiatry* 76 (2005): 1146–51.

11 A. L. Shannon, R. Ferrari, and A. Russell, "Alberta Rodeo Athletes Do Not Develop the Chronic Whiplash Syndrome," *J Rheumatol* 33 (2006): 975–77.

12 H. Malik and M. Lovell, "Soft Tissue Neck Symptoms following High-Energy Road Traffic Accidents," *Spine* 29 (2004): E315–17.

13 J. A. Dufton, J. A. Kopec, H. Wong, J. D. Cassidy, J. Quon, G. McIntosh, and M. Keohoom, "Prognostic Factors Associated with Minimal Improvement following Acute Whiplash-Associated Disorders," *Spine* 31 (2006): E759–65.

14 P. Côté, S. Hogg-Johnson, J. D. Cassidy, C. Carroll, J. W. Frank, and C. Bombardier, "Early Aggressive Care and Delayed Recovery from Whiplash: Isolated Finding or Reproducible Result?," *Arthritis Rheum (Arthritis Care Res)* 57 (2007): 861–68.

15 L. Holm, L. J. Carroll, J. D. Cassidy, E. Skillgate, and A. Ahlbom, "Widespread Pain following Whiplash-Associated Disorders: Incidence, Course, and Risk Factors," *J Rheumatol* 34 (2007): 193–200; L. J. Carroll, J. D. Cassidy, and P. Côté, "The Role of Pain Coping Strategies in Prognosis after Whiplash Injury: Passive Coping Predicts Slowed Recovery," *Pain* 124 (2006): 18–26.

16 N. J. Wiles, G. T. Jones, A. J. Silman, and G. J. Macfarlane, "Onset of Neck Pain after a Motor Vehicle Accident: A Case-Control Study," *J Rheumatol* 32 (2005): 1576–83.

17 R. J. Brison, L. Harting, S. Dostaler, A. Leger, B. H. Rowe, I. Stiell, and W. Pickett, "A Randomized Controlled Trial of an Educational Intervention to Prevent the Chronic Pain of Whiplash Associated Disorders following Rear-End Motor Vehicle Collisions," *Spine* 30 (2005): 1799–1807.

18 A. P. Verhagen, G. G. M. Peeters, R. A. de Bie, and R. A. B. Oostendorp, "Conservative Treatment for Whiplash," Cochrane Library, 4 (Oxford: Update Software, 2001).

19 J. D. Cassidy, L. J. Carroll, P. Côté, and J. Frank, "Does Multidisciplinary Rehabilitation Benefit Whiplash Recovery?," *Spine* 32 (2007): 126–31.

20 J. Kaptchuk, W. B. Stason, R. B. Davis, A. T. R. Legedza, R. N. Schnyer, C. E. Kerr, D. A. Stone, B. H. Nam, I. Kirsch, and R. H. Goldman, "Sham Device v. Inert Pill: Randomised Controlled Trial of Two Placebo Treatments," *BMJ* 332 (2006): 391–97.

21 Y. Lucire, *Constructing RSI: Belief and Desire* (Sydney: University of New South Wales Press, 2003); N. M. Hadler, *Occupational Musculoskeletal Disorders*, 3rd ed. (Philadelphia: Lippincott Williams & Wilkins, 2005).

22 N. Gevitz, ed., *Other Healers: Unorthodox Medicine in America* (Baltimore: Johns Hopkins University Press, 1988), p. 11.

23 H. C. Sox, "Medical Professionalism and the Parable of the Craft Guilds," *Ann Intern Med* 147 (2007): 809–10.

24 M. C. P. Livingston, "Spinal Manipulation in Medical Practice: A Century of Ignorance," *Medical Journal of Australia* 2 (1968): 552–55.

25 J. D. Howell, "The Paradox of Osteopathy," *N Engl J Med* 341 (1999): 1965–68.

26 P. G. Shakelle, "What Role for the Chiropractic in Health Care?," *N Engl J Med* 339 (1998): 1074–75.

27 J. Balen, P. D. Aker, E. R. Crowther, C. Danielson, P. G. Cox, D. O'Shaughnessy, C. Walker, C. H. Goldsmith, E. Duku, and M. R. Sears, "A Comparison of Active and Stimulated Chiropractic Manipulation as Adjunctive Treatment for Childhood Asthma," *N Engl J Med* 339 (1998): 1013–20.

28 N. M. Hadler, P. Curtis, D. B. Gillings, and S. Stinnett, "A Benefit of Spinal Manipulation as Adjunctive Therapy for Acute Low Back Pain: A Stratified Controlled Trial," *Spine* 12 (1987): 703–6.

29 G. B. J. Andersson, T. Lucente, A. M. Davis, R. E. Kappler, J. A. Lipton, and S. Leurgans, "A Comparison of Osteopathic Spinal Manipulation with Standard Care for Patients with Low Back Pain," *N Engl J Med* 341 (1999): 1426–31; J. C. Licciardone, S. T. Stoll, K. G. Fulda, D. P. Russo, J. Siu, W. Winn, and J. Swift, "Osteopathic Manipulative Treatment for Chronic Low Back Pain," *Spine* 28 (2003): 1355–62.

30 W. J. J. Assendelft, S. C. Morton, E. I. Yu, M. J. Suttorp, and P. G. Shekelle, "Spinal Manipulative Therapy for Low Back Pain: A Meta-Analysis of Effectiveness Relative to Other Therapies," *Ann Intern Med* 138 (2003): 871–81.

31 R. A. Deyo, "Treatments for Back Pain: Can We Get Past Trivial Effects?," *Ann Intern Med* 141 (2004): 957–58.

32 T. S. Carey, J. Garrett, A. Jackman, C. McLaughlin, J. Fryer, D. R. Smucker, and the N.C. Back Pain Project, "The Outcomes and Costs of Care for Acute Low Back Pain among Patients Seen by Primary Care Practitioners, Chiropractors, and Orthopedic Surgeons," *N Engl J Med* 333 (1995): 913–17.

33 E. L. Hurwitz, H. Morgenstern, and F. Yu, "Satisfaction as a Predictor of Clinical Outcomes among Chiropractic and Medical Patients Enrolled in the UCLA Low Back Pain Study," *Spine* 30 (2005): 2121–28.

34 R. P. Hertzman-Miller, H. Morgenstern, E. L. Hurwitz, F. Yu, A. H. Adams, P. Harber, and G. F. Kominski, "Comparing the Satisfaction of Low Back Pain Patients Randomized to Receive Medical or Chiropractic Care: Results from the UCLA Low Back Pain Study," *American Journal of Public Health* 92 (2002): 1628–33.

35 UK BEAM Trial Team, "United Kingdom Back Pain Exercise and Manipulation (UK BEAM) Randomised Trial: Effectiveness of Physical Treatments for Back Pain in Primary Care," *BMJ* 329 (2004): 1377–81; D. M. Eisenberg, D. E. Post, R. B.

Davis, M. T. Connelly, A. T. R. Legedza, A. L. Hrbek, L. A. Prosser, J. E. Buring, T. S. Inui, and D. C. Cherkin, "Addition of Choice of Complementary Therapies to Usual Care for Acute Low Back Pain," *Spine* 32 (2007): 151–58.

36 E. L. Hurwitz, H. Morgenstern, G. F. Kominski, F. Yu, and L.-M. Chiang, "A Randomized Trial of Chiropractic and Medical Care for Patients with Low Back Pain," *Spine* 31 (2006): 611–21.

37 J. A. Austin, "Why Patients Use Alternative Medicine," *JAMA* 279 (1998): 1548–53.

38 I. D. Coulter, E. L. Hurwitz, A. H. Adams, B. J. Genovese, R. Hays, and P. G. Shekelle, "Patients Using Chiropractors in North America: Who Are They, and Why Are They in Chiropractic Care?," *Spine* 27 (2002): 291–97.

39 A. K. Burton, T. D. McClune, R. D. Clarke, and C. J. Main, "Long-Term Follow-up of Patients with Low Back Pain Attending for Manipulative Care: Outcomes and Predictors," *Manual Therapy* 9 (2004): 30–35.

40 R. A. Deyo, S. Mirza, and B. I. Martin, "Back Pain Prevalence and Visit Rates: Estimates from U.S. National Surveys, 2002," *Spine* 31 (2006): 2724–27.

41 P. Enthoven, E. Skargren, and B. Oberg, "Clinical Course in Patients Seeking Primary Care for Back or Neck Pain: A Prospective 5-Year Follow-up of Outcome and Health Care Consumption with Subgroup Analysis," *Spine* 29 (2004): 2458–65.

Chapter Six

1 J. T. Goodrich, "History of Spine Surgery in the Ancient and Medieval Worlds," *Neurosurgical Focus* 16, no. 1 (2004): 1–13.

2 R. Dallek, "The Medical Ordeals of JFK," *Atlantic Monthly*, December 2002.

3 1976 Medical Device Amendments, 21 U.S.C. § 301 et. seq. to the Federal Food, Drug, and Cosmetic Act, 21 U.S.C. § 301 et. seq.

4 *Medtronic, Inc. v. Lohr*, 518 U.S. 470 (1996).

5 G. D. Curfman, S. Morrissey, and J. M. Drazen, "A Pivotal Medical-Device Case," *N Engl J Med* 358 (2008): 76–77.

6 P. R. Schwetschenau, A. Ramirez, J. Johnston, C. Wiggs, and A. N. Martins, "Double-Blind Evaluation of Intradiscal Chymopapain for Herniated Lumbar Discs: Early Results," *Journal of Neurosurgery* 45 (1976): 622–27.

7 "Chymopapain Approved," FDA *Drug Bulletin* 12 (1982): 61–63.

8 J. S. Saal and J. A. Saal, "Management of Chronic Discogenic Low Back Pain with a Thermal Intradiscal Catheter: A Preliminary Report," *Spine* 25 (2000): 382–88.

9 J. A. Saal and J. S. Saal, "Intradiscal Electrothermal Treatment for Chronic Discogenic Low Back Pain: A Prospective Outcome Study with Minimum 1-Year Follow-up," *Spine* 25 (2000): 262–67.

10 J. A. Saal and J. S. Saal, "Intradiscal Electrothermal Treatment for Chronic Discogenic Low Back Pain: A Prospective Outcome Study with Minimum 2-Year Follow-up," *Spine* 27 (2002): 966–74.

11 M. Karasek and N. Bogduk, "Twelve-Month Follow-up of a Controlled Trial of Intradiscal Thermal Anuloplasty for Back Pain due to Internal Disc Disruption," *Spine* 25 (2000): 2601–7.

12 B. J. C. Freeman, R. D. Fraser, C. M. J. Cain, D. J. Hall, and D. C. L. Chapple, "A Randomized, Double-Blind Controlled Trial: Intradiscal Electrothermal Therapy versus Placebo for the Treatment of Chronic Discogenic Low Back Pain," *Spine* 30 (2005): 2369–77.

13 R. Derby, R. M. Baker, C.-H. Lee, and P. A. Anderson, "Evidence-Informed Management of Chronic Low Back Pain with Intradiscal Electrothermal Therapy," *Spine Journal* 8 (2008): 80–95.

14 G. Onik, J. Maroon, C. Helms, J. Schweigel, V. Mooney, N. Kahanovitz, A. Day, J. Morris, J. A. McCulloch, and M. Reicher, "Automated Percutaneous Discectomy: Initial Patient Experience," *Radiology* 162 (1987): 129–32.

15 G. Onik and C. A. Helms, "Automated Percutaneous Lumbar Discectomy," *American Journal of Roentgenology* 156 (1991): 531–38.

16 M. Revel, C. Payan, C. Vallee, J. D. Laredo, B. Lassale, C. Roux, H. Carter, C. Salomon, E. Delmas, and others, "Automated Percutaneous Lumbar Discectomy versus Chemonucleolysis in the Treatment of Sciatica: A Randomized Multicenter Trial," *Spine* 18 (1993): 1–7.

17 N. M. Hadler, *Worried Sick: A Prescription for Health in an Overtreated America* (Chapel Hill: University of North Carolina Press, 2008).

18 L. L. Wiltse, "The History of Spinal Disorders," in *The Adult Spine*, 2nd ed., ed. J. W. Frymoyer, T. B. Ducker, N. M. Hadler, and others (Philadelphia: Lippincott-Raven, 1997), pp. 3–40.

19 H. F. Farfan, "The Effects of Torsion of the Intervertebral Joints," *Canadian Journal of Surgery* 12 (1969): 336–41.

20 J. G. Love, "Removal of Intervertebral Discs without Laminectomy," *Mayo Clinic Proceedings* 14 (1939): 800–805.

21 R. W. Williams, "Microsurgical Lumbar Discectomy," *Neurosurgery* 4 (1979): 130–35.

22 E. J. Carragee, S. J. Paragioudakis, and S. Khurana, "Lumbar High-Intensity Zone and Discography in Subjects without Low Back Problems," *Spine* 25 (2000): 2987–92.

23 E. J. Carragee, T. Lincoln, V. S. Parmar, and T. Alamin, "A Gold Standard Evaluation of the 'Discogenic Pain' Diagnosis as Determined by Provocative Discography," *Spine* 31 (2006): 2115–23.

24 G. E. Ehrlich, "Low Back Pain," *Bulletin of the World Health Organization* 81 (2003): 671–76.

25 J. N. Weinstein, J. D. Lurie, P. R. Olson, K. K. Bronner, and E. S. Fisher, "United States' Trends and Regional Variations in Lumbar Spine Surgery: 1992–2003," *Spine* 31 (2006): 2707–14.

26 J. N. Weinstein and J. D. Birkmeyer, eds., *The Dartmouth Atlas of Musculoskeletal Health Care* (Chicago: American Hospital Association Press, 2000).

27 H. Weber, "Lumbar Disc Herniation: A Controlled, Prospective Study with Ten Years of Observation," *Spine* 8 (1983): 131–40.

28 A. Nachemson, "Lumbar Disc Disease with Discogenic Pain: What Surgical Treatment Is Most Effective? Never Treat with Surgery," *Spine* 21 (1996): 1835–36.

29 H. Österman, S. Seitsalo, J. Karppinen, and A. Malmivaara, "Effectiveness of

Microdiscectomy for Lumbar Disc Herniation: A Randomized Controlled Trial with 2 Years of Follow-up," *Spine* 31 (2006): 2409–14.

30 W. C. Peul, H. C. van Houwelingen, W. B. van den Hout, R. Brand, J. A. H. Eekhof, J. T. J. Tans, T. W. M. Thomeer, and B. W. Koes for the Leiden–The Hague Spine Intervention Prognostic Study Group, "Surgery versus Prolonged Conservative Therapy for Sciatica," *N Engl J Med* 356 (2007): 2245–56.

31 J. N. Weinstein, T. D. Tosteson, J. D. Lurie, A. N. A. Tosteson, B. Hanscom, J. S. Skiner, W. A. Abdu, A. S. Hilibrand, S. D. Boden, and R. A. Deyo, "Surgical vs. Non-operative Treatment for Lumbar Disk Herniation," *JAMA* 296 (2006): 2441–50.

32 J. N. Weinstein, J. D. Lurie, T. D. Tosteson, A. N. A. Tosteson, E. A. Blood, W. A. Abdu, H. Herkowitz, A. Hilbrand, T. Albert, and J. Fischgrund, "Surgical versus Nonoperative Treatment for Lumbar Disc Herniation: Four-Year Results for the Spine Patient Outcomes Research Trial (SPORT)," *Spine* 33 (2008): 2789–800.

33 T. Hansson, E. Hansson, and H. Malchau, "Utility of Spine Surgery: A Comparison of Common Elective Orthopaedic Surgical Procedures," *Spine* 33 (2008): 2819–30.

34 A. F. DePalma and R. H. Rothman, "The Nature of Pseudoarthrosis," *Clinical Orthopedics and Related Research* 59 (1968): 113–18.

35 J. W. Frymoyer, E. Hanley, J. Howe, D. Kuhlmann, and R. Matteri, "Disc Excision and Spine Fusion in the Management of Lumbar Disc Disease: A Minimum Ten Year Follow-up," *Spine* 3 (1978): 1–6.

36 R. A. Hart, "Failed Spine Surgery Syndrome in the Life and Career of John Fitzgerald Kennedy," *Journal of Bone and Joint Surgery* (American) 88 (2006): 1141–48.

37 R. Roy-Camille, G. Saillant, and C. Mazel, "Internal Fixation of the Lumbar Spine with Pedicle Screw Plating," *Clinical Orthopedics and Related Research* 203 (1986): 7–17.

38 R. A. Deyo, D. T. Grat, W. Kreuter, S. Mirza, and B. I. Martin, "United States Trends in Lumbar Fusion Surgery for Degenerative Conditions," *Spine* 30 (2005): 1441–45.

39 R. V. Shah, T. J. Albert, V. Breugel-Sanchez, A. R. Vaccaro, A. S. Hilibrand, and J. N. Brauer, "Industry Support and Correlation to Study Outcome for Papers Published in *Spine*," *Spine* 30 (2005): 1099–104.

40 P. Fritzell, O. Hägg, P. Wessberg, A. Nordwall, and the Swedish Lumbar Spine Study Group, "Lumbar Fusion versus Nonsurgical Treatment for Chronic Low Back Pain," *Spine* 26 (2001): 2521–34.

41 B. Kwon, J. N. Katz, D. H. Kim, and L. G. Jenis, "A Review of the 2001 Volvo Award Winner in Clinical Studies; Lumbar Fusion versus Nonsurgical Treatment for Chronic Low Back Pain: A Multicenter Randomized Controlled Trial from the Swedish Lumbar Spine Study Group," *Spine* 31 (2006): 245–49.

42 J. I. Brox, R. Sørensen, A. Friis, Ø. Nygaard, A. Indahl, A. Keller, T. Ingebrigtsen, H. R. Eriksen, I. Holm, A. K. Koller, R. Riise, and O. Reiderås, "Randomized Clinical Trial of Lumbar Instrumented Fusion and Cognitive Intervention and Exercises in Patients with Chronic Low Back Pain and Disc Degeneration," *Spine* 28 (2003): 1913–21.

43 J. Fairbank, H. Frost, J. Wilson-MacDonald, L.-M. Yu, K. Barker, and R. Collins for the Spine Stabilisation Trial Group, "Randomised Controlled Trial to Compare Surgical Stabilization of the Lumbar Spine with an Intensive Rehabilitation Programme for Patients with Chronic Low Back Pain: The MRC Spine Stabilization Trial," *BMJ* 330 (2005): 1233–39.

44 R. A. Deyo, A. Nachemson, and S. K. Mirza, "Spinal-Fusion Surgery—The Case for Restraint," *N Engl J Med* 350 (2004): 722–26; B. W. Koes, "Surgery versus Intensive Rehabilitation Programmes for Chronic Low Back Pain: Spinal Fusion Surgery Has Only Modest, if Any, Effects," *BMJ* 330 (2005): 1220–21; E. Carragee, "Surgical Treatment of Lumbar Disk Disorders," *JAMA* 296 (2006): 2485–87; R. A. Deyo, "Back Surgery—Who Needs It?," *N Engl J Med* 356 (2007): 2239–43.

45 J. N. A. Gibson and G. Waddell, "Surgical Interventions for Lumbar Disc Prolapse," Updated Cochrane Review, *Spine* 32 (2007): 1735–47; J. N. A. Gibson and G. Waddell, "Surgical Interventions for Lumbar Disc Prolapse," Cochrane Database of Systematic Reviews (2007), issue 2, art. no. CD001350, DOI: 10.1002/14651858. CD001350.pub4.

46 R. Abelson, "The Spine as a Profit Center," *New York Times*, December 30, 2006.

47 N. M. Hadler and the Ethics Forum, "Would Physician Disclosure of All Industry Gifts Solve the Conflict-of-Interest Problem? Negative Constructive," *American Medical News*, January 7, 2008.

48 J. Mitchell, "Utilization Changes following Market Entry by Physician-Owned Specialty Hospitals," *Medical Care Research and Review* 64 (2007): 395–415.

49 J. L. Zeller, "Artificial Spinal Disk Superior to Fusion for Treating Degenerative Disk Disease," *JAMA* 296 (2006): 2665–67.

50 J. Zigler, R. Delamarter, J. M. Spivak, R. J. Linovitz, G. O. Danielson, T. T. Haider, F. Cammisa, J. Zuchermann, R. Balderston, S. Kitchel, K. Foley, R. Watkins, D. Bradford, J. Yue, H. Yuan, H. Herkowitz, D. Geiger, J. Bendo, T. Peppers, B. Sachs, F. Girardi, M. Kropf, and J. Goldstein, "Results of the Prospective, Randomized, Multicenter Food and Drug Administration Investigational Device Exemption Study of the ProDisc-L Total Disc Replacement versus Circumferential Fusion for Treatment of 1-Level Degenerative Disc Disease," *Spine* 32 (2007): 1155–62.

51 J. Zigler, J. Walsh, and J. Zigler, "Medical Device Reporting: Issues with Class III Medical Devices," *Food and Drug Law Journal* 62 (2007): 573–80.

52 R. Abelson, "Financial Ties Are Cited as Issue in Spine Study," *New York Times*, January 30, 2008.

Chapter Seven

1 J. Barry and C. Jones, eds., *Medicine and Charity before the Welfare State* (London: Routledge, 1991).

2 W. I. Trattner, *From Poor Law to Welfare State* (New York: Free Press, 1994).

3 C. E. Rosenberg, *The Care of Strangers: The Rise of America's Hospital System* (New York: Basic Books, 1987), p. 322.

4 G. Orwell, "How the Poor Die," in *The Orwell Reader* (New York: Harcourt Brace, 1984), pp. 89–95.

5 J. London, *The People of the Abyss*, in *Jack London: Novels and Social Writings* (New York: Library Classics of the United States, 1982), p. 165.

6 H. Mayhew, *London Labour and the London Poor*, vols. 1–4 (New York: Dover Publications, 1968).

7 J. Grigg, *Lloyd George: The People's Champion, 1902–1911* (London: Eyre Methuen, 1978), p. 333.

8 H. M. Somers and A. R. Somers, *Workmen's Compensation* (New York: Wiley, 1954), p. 18.

9 G. A. Craig, *Germany, 1866–1945* (Oxford: Oxford University Press, 1978), pp. 150–52.

10 H. Beck, *The Origins of the Authoritarian Welfare State in Prussia* (Ann Arbor: University of Michigan Press, 1995), p. 241.

11 M. Savage and A. Miles, *The Remaking of the British Working Class, 1840–1940* (London: Routledge, 1994), pp. 50–55.

12 N. M. Hadler, "The Disabling Backache: An International Perspective," *Spine* 20 (1995): 640–49.

13 R. H. Cox, *The Development of the Dutch Welfare State* (Pittsburgh: University of Pittsburgh Press, 1993).

14 T. Billroth, *The Medical Sciences in the German Universities: A Study in the History of Civilization* (New York: Macmillan, 1924), p. 91.

15 I. M. Rubinow, *Social Insurance* (New York: Henry Holt, 1916).

16 J. L. Kreader, "Isaac Max Rubinow: Pioneering Specialist in Social Insurance," *Social Service Review* 50 (1976): 402–25.

17 I. M. Rubinow, *The Quest for Security* (New York: Henry Holt, 1934), pp. 20–21.

18 T. F. Schlabach, *Edwin E. Witte: Cautious Reformer* (Madison: State Historical Society of Wisconsin, 1969).

19 E. E. Wittee, *The Development of the Social Security Act* (Madison: University of Wisconsin Press, 1963).

20 N. M. Hadler, "Legal Ramifications of the Medical Definition of Back Disease," *Ann Intern Med* 89 (1978): 992–99.

21 N. M. Hadler, "Workers' Compensation and Chronic Regional Musculoskeletal Pain," *British Journal of Rheumatology* 37 (1998): 815–18.

22 A. E. Dembe, *Occupation and Disease* (New Haven: Yale University Press, 1996), pp. 24–101.

23 W. J. Mixter and J. S. Barr, "Rupture of the Intervertebral Disc with Involvement of the Spinal Canal," *N Engl J Med* 211 (1934): 210–15.

24 W. J. Mixter and J. B. Ayer, "Herniation or Rupture of the Intervertebral Disc into the Spinal Canal," *N Engl J Med* 213 (1935): 385–95.

25 M. C. Battié, T. Videman, and E. Parent, "Lumbar Disc Degeneration: Epidemiology and Genetic Influences," *Spine* 29 (2004): 2679–90; T. Videman, M. C. Battié, S. Ripatti, K. Gill, H. Manninen, and J. Kaprio, "Determinants of the Progression in Lumbar Degeneration: A 5-Year Follow-up Study of Adult Male Monozygotic

Twins," *Spine* 31 (2006): 671–78; M. C. Battié, T. Videman, J. Kaprio, and others, "The Twin Spine Study: Contributions to a Changing View of Disc Degeneration," *Spine Journal* 9 (2009): 47–59.

26 N. M. Hadler, "MRI for Regional Back Pain: Need for Less Imaging, Better Understanding," *JAMA* 289 (2003): 2863–65.

27 K. P. Martimo, J. Verbeek, J. Karppinen, A. D. Furland, P. P. R. M. Kuijer, E. Viidari-Juntura, E. P. Takala, and M. Jauhiainen, "Manual Material Handling Advice and Assistive Devices for Preventing and Treating Back Pain in Workers" (review), Cochrane Database of Systematic Reviews (2007), issue 3, art. no. CD005958, DOI: 10.1002/14651858.CD005958.pub2.

28 E. Carragee, T. Alamin, I. Cheng, T. Franklin, and E. Hurwitz, "Does Minor Trauma Cause Serious Low Back Illness?," *Spine* 31 (2006): 2942–49.

29 N. M. Hadler, *Occupational Musculoskeletal Disorders*, 3rd ed. (Philadelphia: Lippincott Williams & Wilkins, 2005).

30 L. Hashemi, B. S. Webster, and E. A. Clancy, "Trends in Disability Duration and Costs of Workers' Compensation Low Back Pain Claims (1988–1996)," *J Occup Environ Med* 40 (1998): 110–19.

31 F. Blum and J. F. Burton, "Workers' Compensation Costs in 2005: Regional, Industrial, and Other Variations," *Workers' Compensation Policy Review* 6, no. 4 (2006): 3–20.

32 E. R. Tichauer, "Some Aspects of Stress on Forearm and Hand in Industry," *Journal of Occupational Medicine* 8 (1966): 63–71.

33 S. H. Snook, C. H. Irvine, and S. F. Bass, "Maximum Weight and Work Loads Acceptable to Male Industrial Workers," *American Industrial Hygiene Association Journal* 31 (1970): 579–86.

34 D. B. Chaffin and K. S. Park, "A Longitudinal Study of Low-Back Pain as Associated with Occupational Weight Lifting Factors," *American Industrial Hygiene Association Journal* 34 (1973): 513–25; D. B. Chaffin, "Human Strength Capability and Low-Back Pain," *Journal of Occupational Medicine* 16 (1974): 248–54.

35 S. A. Lavender, D. M. Oleske, L. Nicholson, G. B. Andersson, and J. Hahn, "Comparison of Five Methods Used to Determine Low Back Disorder Risk in a Manufacturing Environment," *Spine* 24 (1999): 1441–48.

36 N. G. Stillman and J. R. Wheeler, "The Expansion of Occupational Safety and Health Law," *Notre Dame Law Review* 62 (1987): 969–1009.

37 B. P. Bernard, ed., *Musculoskeletal Disorders and Workplace Factors*, DHHS (NIOSH) Publication no. 97–141 (Cincinnati: NIOSH, 1997).

38 R. J. Gatchel and D. C. Turk, "Criticisms of the Biopsychosocial Model in Spine Care," *Spine* 25 (2008): 2831–36.

39 I. A. Harris, J. M. Young, H. Rae, B. B. Jalaludin, and M. J. Solomon, "Factors Associated with Back Pain after Physical Injury: A Survey of Consecutive Major Trauma Patients," *Spine* 32 (2007): 1561–65.

40 R. A. Deyo, S. K. Mirza, and B. I. Martin, "Back Pain Prevalence and Visit Rates," *Spine* 31 (2006): 2724–27.

41 L. H. M. Pengel, R. D. Herbert, C. G. Maher, and K. M. Refshauge, "Acute Low Back Pain: Systematic Review of Its Prognosis," *BMJ* 327 (2003): 323–27.

42 J. M. Hush, K. Refshauge, G. Sullivan, L. de Souza, C. G. Maher, and J. H. McAuley, "Recovery: What Does This Mean to Patients with Low Back Pain?," *Arthritis Rheum (Arthritis Care Res)* 61 (2009): 124–31.

43 T. R. Stanton, N. Henschke, C. G. Maher, K. M. Refshauge, J. Latimer, and J. H. McAuley, "After an Episode of Acute Low Back Pain, Recurrence Is Unpredictable and Not as Common as Previously Thought," *Spine* 33 (2008): 2923–28.

44 A. Magora, "Investigation of the Relation between Low Back Pain and Occupation: V. Psychological Aspects," *Scandinavian Journal of Rehabilitation Medicine* 5 (1973): 191–96.

45 N. M. Hadler, "The Injured Worker and the Internist," *Ann Intern Med* 120 (1994): 163–64.

46 S. J. Linton, "A Review of Psychological Risk Factors in Back and Neck Pain," *Spine* 25 (2000): 1148–56; W. E. Hoogendoorn, N. M. van Popper, P. M. Bongers, B. W. Koes, and L. M. Bouter, "Systematic Review of Psychosocial Factors at Work and Private Life as Risk Factors for Back Pain," *Spine* 25 (2000): 2114–25.

47 E. F. Harkness, G. J. Macfarlane, E. S. Nahit, A. J. Silman, and J. McBeth, "Risk Factors for New-Onset Low Back Pain amongst Cohorts of Newly Employed Workers," *Rheumatology* 42 (2003): 959–68; S. Bartys, K. Burton, and C. Main, "A Prospective Study of Psychosocial Risk Factors and Absence due to Musculoskeletal Disorders—Implications for Occupational Screening," *Occupational Medicine* 55 (2005): 375–79.

48 E. Clays, D. de Bacquer, F. Leynen, M. Kornitzer, F. Kittel, and G. de Backer, "The Impact of Psychosocial Factors on Low Back Pain: Longitudinal Results from the Belstress Study," *Spine* 32 (2007): 262–68.

49 J. Head, M. Kivimäki, P. Martikainen, J. Vahtera, J. E. Ferrie, and M. G. Marmot, "Influence of Change in Psychosocial Work Characteristics on Sickness Absence: The Whitehall II Study," *Journal of Epidemiology and Community Health* 60 (2006): 55–61.

50 F. Lötters, R.-L. Franche, S. Hogg-Johnson, A. Burdorf, and J. D. Pole, "The Prognostic Value of Depressive Symptoms, Fear-Avoidance, and Self-Efficacy for Duration of Lost-Time Benefits in Workers with Musculoskeletal Disorders," *Occup Environ Med* 63 (2006): 794–801.

51 L. Kaila-Kangas, M. Kivimäki, H. Riihimäki, R. Luukkonen, J. Kirjonen, and P. Leino-Arjas, "Psychosocial Factors at Work as Predictors of Hospitalization for Back Disorders: A 28-Year Follow-up of Industrial Employees," *Spine* 29 (2004): 1823–30.

52 M. L. Nielsen, R. Rugulies, K. B. Christensen, L. Smith-Hansen, and T. S. Kristensen, "Psychosocial Work Environment Predictors of Short and Long Spells of Registered Sickness Absence during a 2-Year Follow Up," *J Occup Environ Med* 48 (2006): 591–98.

53 M. Feuerstein, C. B. Harrington, M. Lopez, and A. Haufler, "How Do Job Stress

and Ergonomic Factors Impact Clinic Visits in Acute Low Back Pain? A Prospective Study," *J Occup Environ Med* 48 (2006): 607–14.

54 J. H. Andersen, J. P. Haahr, and P. Frost, "Risk Factors for More Severe Regional Musculoskeletal Symptoms: A Two-Year Prospective Study of a General Working Population," *Arthritis Rheum* 56 (2007): 1355–64.

55 R. A. Lles, M. Davidson, and N. F. Taylor, "Psychosocial Predictors of Failure to Return to Work in Non-chronic Non-specific Low Back Pain: A Systematic Review," *Occup Environ Med* 65 (2008): 507–17.

56 K.-P. Martimo, J. Verbeek, J. Karppinen, A. D. Furlan, E.-P. Takata, P. P. F. M. Kuijer, M. Jauhlainen, and E. Viikari-Juntura, "Effect of Training and Lifting Equipment for Preventing Back Pain in Lifting and Handling: Systematic Review," *BMJ* 336 (2008): 429–31.

57 DoD Ergonomics Working Group, "Psychosocial Factors and Musculoskeletal Disorders," *DoD Ergonomics Working Group News* (⟨www.ergoworkinggroup.org⟩), issue 72 (2007): 1–2.

58 N. M. Hadler, "Comments on the 'Ergonomics Program Standard' Proposed by the Occupational Safety and Health Administration," *J Occup Environ Med* 42 (2000): 951–69.

59 R. J. Butler, W. G. Johnson, and P. Côté, "It Pays to Be Nice: Employer-Worker Relationships and the Management of Back Pain Claims," *J Occup Environ Med* 49 (2007): 214–25.

60 T. J. Mielenz, J. M. Garrett, and T. S. Carey, "Association of Psychosocial Work Characteristics with Low Back Pain Outcomes," *Spine* 33 (2008): 1270–75.

61 N. M. Hadler, "Rheumatology and the Health of the Workforce," *Arthritis Rheum* 44 (2001): 1971–74.

62 R. C. Tait, J. T. Chibnall, E. M. Andresen, and N. M. Hadler, "Management of Occupational Back Injuries: Differences among African Americans and Caucasians," *Pain* 112 (2004): 389–96.

63 J. T. Chibnall, R. C. Tait, E. M. Andresen, and N. M. Hadler, "Race Differences in Diagnosis and Surgery for Occupational Low Back Injuries," *Spine* 31 (2006): 1272–75; I. Harris, J. Mulford, M. Solomon, J. M. van Gelder, and J. Young, "Association between Compensation Status and Outcome after Surgery: A Meta-Analysis," *JAMA* 293 (2005): 1644–52.

64 R. C. Tait, J. T. Chibnall, E. M. Andresen, and N. M. Hadler, "Disability Determination: Validity with Occupational Low Back Pain," *Journal of Pain* 7 (2006): 951–57.

65 N. M. Hadler, "Workers with Disabling Back Pain," *N Engl J Med* 337 (1997): 341–43.

Chapter Eight

1 T. S. Carey, A. Evans, N. Hadler, W. Kalsbeek, C. McLaughlin, and J. Fryer, "Care-Seeking among Individuals with Chronic Low Back Pain," *Spine* 20 (1995): 312–17; J. K. Freburger, G. M. Holmes, R. P. Agans, and others, "The Rising Prevalence of Low Back Pain," *Archives of Internal Medicine* 169 (2009): 251–58.

2 T. S. Carey, J. M. Garrett, A. Jackman, N. M. Hadler, and the North Carolina Back Pain Project, "Recurrence and Care Seeking after Acute Back Pain: Results of a Long-Term Follow-up Study," *Medical Care* 37 (1999): 157–64.

3 N. M. Hadler, T. S. Carey, and J. Garrett, "The Influence of Indemnification by Workers' Compensation Insurance on Recovery from Acute Backache," *Spine* 20 (1995): 2710–15.

4 K. M. Dunn, K. Jordan, and P. R. Croft, "Characterizing the Course of Low Back Pain: A Latent Class Analysis," *American Journal of Epidemiology* 163 (2006): 754–61.

5 J. D. Cassidy, P. Côté, L. J. Carroll, and V. Kristman, "Incidence and Course of Low Back Pain Episodes in the General Population," *Spine* 30 (2005): 2817–23.

6 N. M. Hadler and T. S. Carey, "Low Back Pain: An Intermittent and Remittent Predicament of Life," *Ann Rheum Dis* 57 (1998): 1–2.

7 C. Chen, S. Hogg-Johnson, and P. Smith, "The Recovery Patterns of Back Pain among Workers with Compensated Occupational Back Injuries," *Occup Environ Med* 64 (2007): 534–40.

8 N. M. Hadler, "Back Pain in the Workplace: What You Lift or How You Lift Matters Far Less than Whether You Lift or When," *Spine* 22 (1997): 935–40.

9 J. M. Melhorn and W. E. Ackerman, eds., *Guides to the Evaluation of Disease and Injury Causation* (Chicago: American Medical Association, 2008), pp. 114–29.

10 T. K. Courtney, S. Matz, and B. S. Webster, "Disabling Occupational Injury in the U.S. Construction Industry, 1996," *J Occup Environ Med* 44 (2002): 1161–68.

11 I. Sengupta, V. Reno, and J. F. Burton, *Workers' Compensation: Benefits, Coverage, and Costs, 2005* (Washington, D.C.: National Academy of Social Insurance, 2007), pp. 1–94.

12 C. Rasmussen, C. Leboeuf-Yde, L. Hestbæk, and C. Manniche, "Poor Outcome in Patients with Spine-Related Leg or Arm Pain Who Are Involved in Compensation Claims: A Prospective Study of Patients in the Secondary Care Sector," *Scandinavian Journal of Rheumatology* 37 (2008): 462–68; E. J. Bernacki and X. Tao, "The Relationship between Attorney Involvement, Claim Duration and Worker's Compensation Costs," *J Occup Environ Med* 50 (2008): 1013–18.

13 I. D. Cameron, T. Rebbeck, D. Sindhusake, G. Rubin, A.-M. Feyer, J. Walsh, and W. N. Schofield, "Legislative Change Is Associated with Improved Health Status in People with Whiplash," *Spine* 33 (2008): 250–54.

14 S. Bartys, K. Burton, and C. Main, "A Prospective Study of Psychosocial Risk Factors and Absence due to Musculoskeletal Disorders—Implications for Occupational Screening," *Occupational Medicine* 55 (2005): 375–79.

15 N. M. Hadler, "If You Have to Prove You Are Ill, You Can't Get Well," *Spine* 21 (1996): 2397–400.

16 T. Pincus, S. Vogel, A. K. Burton, R. Santos, and A. P. Field, "Fear Avoidance and Prognosis in Back Pain: A Systematic Review and Synthesis of Current Evidence," *Arthritis Rheum* 54 (2006): 3999–4010.

17 S. Øverland, N. Glozier, M. Henderson, J. G. Mæland, M. Hotopf, and A. Mykletun, "Health Status before, during, and after Disability Pension Award: The Hordaland Health Study," *Occup Environ Med* 65 (2008): 769–73.

18 D. M. Phillips, "JCAHO Pain Management Standards Are Unveiled," *JAMA* 284 (2000): 428.

19 J. J. Liszka-Hackzell and D. P. Martin, "An Analysis of the Relationship between Activity and Pain in Chronic and Acute Low Back Pain," *Anesthesia and Analgesia* 99 (2004): 477–81.

20 J. B. Staal, H. Hlobil, J. W. R. Twisk, T. Smid, A. J. A. Köke, and W. van Mechelen, "Graded Activity for Low Back Pain in Occupational Health Care: A Randomized, Controlled Trial," *Ann Intern Med* 140 (2004): 77–84.

21 J. R. Anema, B. Cuelenaere, A. J. van der Beek, D. L. Knol, H. C. W. de Vet, and W. van Mechelen, "The Effectiveness of Ergonomic Interventions on Return-to-Work after Low Back Pain: A Prospective Two Year Cohort Study in Six Countries on Low Back Pain Patients Sicklisted for 3–4 Months," *Occup Environ Med* 61 (2004): 289–94; E. Haukka, P. Leino-Arjas, E. Viikari-Juntura, E.-P. Takala, A. Malmivaara, L. Hopsu, P. Mutanen, R. Ketola, T. Virtanen, I. Pehkonen, M. Holtari-Leino, J. Nykänen, S. Stenholm, E. Nykyri, and H. Riihimäki, "A Randomised Controlled Trial of whether a Participatory Ergonomics Intervention could Prevent Musculoskeletal Disorders," *Occup Environ Med* 65 (2008): 849–56.

22 E. J. Steele, A. P. Dawson, and J. E. Hiller, "School-Based Interventions for Spinal Pain: A Systematic Review," *Spine* 31 (2006): 226–33.

23 G. Waddell, M. Aylward, and P. Sawney, *Back Pain, Incapacity for Work, Social Security Benefits: An International Literature Review and Analysis* (London: The Royal Society of Medicine Press, 2002), 208–12.

24 K. B. Hagen and O. Thune, "Work Incapacity from Low Back Pain in the General Population," *Spine* 23 (1998): 2091–95.

25 I. B. Scheel, K. B. Hagen, J. Herrin, and others, "Blind Faith? The Effects of Promoting Active Sick Leave for Back Pain Patients," *Spine* 27 (2002): 2734–40.

26 E. M. Hagen, A. Grasdal, and H. R. Eriksen, "Does Early Intervention with a Light Mobilization Program Reduce Long-Term Sick Leave for Low Back Pain? A 3-Year Follow-up Study," *Spine* 28 (2003): 2309–16.

27 K. B. Hagen, K. Tambs, and T. Bjerkedal, "A Prospective Cohort Study of Risk Factors for Disability Retirement because of Back Pain in the General Working Population," *Spine* 27 (2002): 1790–96.

28 E. M. Hagen, E. Svensen, H. R. Eriksen, C. M. Ihlebæk, and H. Ursin, "Comorbid Subjective Health Complaints in Low Back Pain," *Spine* 31 (2006): 1491–95.

29 P. Loisel, L. Abenhaim, P. Durand, J. M. Esdaile, S. Suissa, L. Gosselin, R. Simard, J. Turcotte, and J. Lemaire, "A Population-Based, Randomized Clinical Trial on Back Pain Management," *Spine* 22 (1997): 2911–18.

30 P. Loisel, L. Gosselin, P. Durand, J. Lemaire, S. Poitras, and L. Abenhaim, "Implementation of a Participatory Ergonomics Program in the Rehabilitation of Workers Suffering from Subacute Back Pain," *Applied Ergonomics* 32 (2001): 53–60.

31 S. A. Lavender, E. P. Lorenz, and G. B. Andersson, "Can a New Behaviorally Oriented Training Process to Improve Lifting Technique Prevent Occupationally Related Back Injuries due to Lifting?," *Spine* 32 (2007): 487–94; S. J. Bigos, J. Holland, C. Holland, J. S. Webster, M. Battié, and J. A. Malmgren, "High-Quality

Controlled Trials on Preventive Episodes of Back Problems: Systematic Literature Review in Working-Age Adults," *Spine Journal* 9 (2009): 147–68.

32 S. Brage, I. Sandanger, and J. F. Nygård, "Emotional Distress as a Predictor for Low Back Disability: A Prospective 12-Year Population-Based Study," *Spine* 32 (2007): 269–74.

33 N. M. Hadler, *Worried Sick: A Prescription for Health in an Overtreated America* (Chapel Hill: University of North Carolina Press, 2008); N. M. Hadler, *Occupational Musculoskeletal Disorders*, 3rd ed. (Philadelphia: Lippincott Williams & Wilkins, 2005).

34 J. Dersh, T. G. Mayer, R. J. Gatchel, P. B. Polatin, B. R. Theodore, and E. A. K. Mayer, "Prescription Opioid Dependence Is Associated with Poorer Outcomes in Disabling Spinal Disorders," *Spine* 20 (2008): 2219–27.

35 G. M. Franklin, B. D. Stover, J. A. Turner, D. Fulton-Kehoe, and T. M. Wickizer, "Early Opioid Prescription and Subsequent Disability among Workers with Back Injuries," *Spine* 33 (2008): 199–204.

36 A. D. Furlan, J. A. Sandoval, A. Mailis-Gagnon, and E. Tunks, "Opioids for Chronic Noncancer Pain: A Meta-Analysis of Effectiveness and Side Effects," *Canadian Medical Association Journal* 174 (2006): 1589–94.

37 A. Deshpande, A. Furlan, A. Mailis-Gagnon, S. Atlas, and D. Turk, "Opioids for Chronic Low-Back Pain," Cochrane Database of Systematic Reviews (2007), issue 3, art. no. CD004959, DOI: 10.1002/14651858.CD004959.pub3.

38 B. A. Martell, P. G. O'Connor, R. D. Kerns, W. C. Becker, K. S. Morales, T. R. Kosten, and D. A. Fiellin, "Systematic Review; Opioid Treatment for Chronic Back Pain: Prevalence Efficacy and Association with Addiction," *Ann Intern Med* 146 (2007): 116–27.

39 I. Harris, J. Mulford, M. Solomon, J. M. van Gelder, and J. Young, "Association between Compensation Status and Outcome after Surgery," *JAMA* 293 (2005): 1644–52.

40 I. A. Harris, "Personal Injury Compensation," *ANZ Journal of Surgery* 77 (2007): 606–7.

41 J. T. Chibnall, R. C. Tait, E. M. Andresen, and N. M. Hadler, "Race Differences in Diagnosis and Surgery for Occupational Low Back Injuries," *Spine* 31 (2006): 1272–75.

42 K. Baum, "Independent Medical Examinations: An Expanding Source of Physician Liability," *Ann Intern Med* 142 (2005): 974–78.

43 G. Waddell, J. A. McCulloch, E. Kummel, and R. M. Venner, "Nonorganic Physical Signs in Low-Back Pain," *Spine* 5 (1980): 117–25.

44 J. Richman, P. Green, R. Gervais, L. Flaro, T. Merten, R. Brockhaus, and D. Ranks, "Objective Tests of Symptom Exaggeration in Independent Medical Examinations," *J Occup Environ Med* 48 (2006): 303–11.

45 C. Sun, C. Jin, C. Martin, R. Gerbo, Y. Wang, W. Hu, J. Atkins, and A. Ducatman, "Cost and Outcome Analyses on the Timing of First Independent Medical Evaluation in Patients with Work-Related Lumbosacral Sprain," *J Occup Environ Med* 49 (2007): 1264–68.

46 J. B. Staal, R. de Bie, H. C. W. De Vet, J. Hildebrandt, and P. Nelemans, "Injection Therapy for Subacute and Chronic Low Back Pain," Cochrane Database of Systematic Reviews (2008), issue 3, art. no. CD001824, DOI: 10.1002/14651858. CD001824.pub3.

47 M. W. Heymans, M. W. van Tulder, R. Esmail, C. Bobmardier, and B. W. Koes, "Back Schools for Nonspecific Low Back Pain: A Systematic Review within the Framework of the Cochrane Collaboration Back Review Group," Spine 30 (2005): 2153–63.

48 R. W. J. G. Ostelo, M. W. van Tulder, J. W. S. Vlaeyen, S. J. Linton, S. J. Morley, and W. J. J. Assendelft, "Behavioural Treatment for Chronic Low-Back Pain," Cochrane Database of Systematic Reviews (2005), issue 1, art. no. CD002014, DOI: 10.1002/14651858.CD002014.pub2.

49 Staal, de Bie, De Vet, Hildebrandt, and Nelemans, "Injection Therapy for Subacute and Chronic Low Back Pain."

50 L. Brosseau, S. Milne, V. Robinson, S. Marchand, B. Shea, G. Wells, and P. Tugwell, "Efficacy of the Transcutaneous Electrical Nerve Stimulation for the Treatment of Chronic Low Back Pain: A Meta-Analysis," Spine 27 (2002): 596–603.

51 M. van der Hulst, M. M. R. Vollenbroek-Hutten, and M. J. Ijzerman, "A Systematic Review of Sociodemographic, Physical, and Psychological Predictors of Multidisciplinary Rehabilitation—Or, Back School Treatment Outcome in Patients with Chronic Low Back Pain," Spine 30 (2005): 813–25.

52 K. Karjalainen, A. Malmivaara, M. van Tulder, R. Roine, M. Jauhiainen, H. Hurri, and B. Koes, "Multidisciplinary Biopsychosocial Rehabilitation for Subacute Low-Back Pain among Working Age Adults," Cochrane Database of Systematic Reviews (2003), issue 2, art. no. CD002193, DOI: 10.1002/14651858.CD002193.

53 B. M. Hoffman, R. K. Papas, D. K. Chatkoff, and R. D. Kerns, "Meta-Analysis of Psychological Interventions for Chronic Low Back Pain," Health Psychology 26 (2007): 1–9.

54 S. J. Linton and E. Nordin, "A 5-Year Follow-up Evaluation of the Health and Economic Consequences of an Early Cognitive Behavioral Intervention for Back Pain: A Randomized Controlled Trial," Spine 31 (2006): 853–58.

55 M. Foucault, The Birth of the Clinic: An Archaeology of Medical Perception (New York: Vintage Books, 1975).

56 F. Kafka, The Trial (New York: Knopf, 1956), pp. 217–20.

57 M. Brod, Franz Kafka: A Biography (New York: Schockian, 1947), p. 84.

58 M. Osterweis, A. Kleinman, and D. Mechanic, eds., Pain and Disability (Washington, D.C.: National Academy Press, 1987), pp. 21–36.

59 Ibid., p. 25.

60 T. S. Carey, N. M. Hadler, D. Gillings, S. Stinnett, and T. Wallsten, "Medical Disability Assessment of the Back Pain Patient for the Social Security Administration: The Weighting of Presenting Clinical Features," Journal of Clinical Epidemiology 41 (1988): 691–97.

61 D. H. Autor and M. G. Duggan, "The Growth in the Social Security Disability Rolls: A Fiscal Crisis Unfolding," Journal of Economic Perspectives 29 (2006): 71–96.

62 J. Head, M. Kivimäki, P. Martikainen, J. Vahtera, J. E. Ferrie, and M. G. Marmot, "Influence of Change in Psychosocial Work Characteristics on Sickness Absence: The Whitehall II Study," *Journal of Epidemiology and Community Health* 60 (2006): 55–61.

63 N. M. Hadler, "Backache and Work Incapacity in Japan," *Journal of Occupational Medicine* 36 (1994): 1110–14.

64 Autor and Duggan, "The Growth in the Social Security Disability Rolls."

65 D. C. Stapleton and R. V. Burkhauser, *The Decline in Employment of People with Disabilities: A Policy Puzzle* (Kalamazoo, Mich.: Upjohn Institute for Employment Research, 2003); R. Burkhauser and M. Daly, "Policy Watch: U.S. Disability Policy in a Changing Environment," *Journal of Economic Perspectives* 16 (2002): 213–24.

66 P. Mirowski, "Naturalizing the Market on the Road to Revisionism: Bruce Caldwell's *Hayek's Challenge* and the Challenge of Hayek Interpretation," *Journal of Institutional Economics* 3 (2007): 351–72.

67 R. C. Tait, J. T. Chibnall, E. M. Andresen, and N. M. Hadler, "Disability Determination: Validity with Occupational Low Back Pain," *Journal of Pain* 7 (2006): 951–57.

68 J. T. Chibnall, R. C. Tait, E. M. Andresen, and N. M. Hadler, "Clinical and Social Predictors of Application for Social Security Disability Insurance by Workers' Compensation Claimants with Low Back Pain," *J Occup Environ Med* 48 (2006): 733–40.

69 E. J. Huth, "Illness," in *The Healer's Art: A New Approach to the Doctor-Patient Relationship*, ed. E. Cassell (New York: Lippincott, 1976), p. 48.

70 E. Freidson, *Medical Work in America: Essays on Health Care* (New Haven: Yale University Press, 1989).

71 P. Starr, *The Social Transformation of American Medicine* (New York: Basic Books, 1982).

72 S. H. Ehringhaus, J. S. Weissman, J. L. Sears, S. D. Goold, S. Feibelmann, and E. G. Campbell, "Responses of Medical Schools to Institutional Conflicts of Interest," *JAMA* 299 (2008): 665–71.

73 K. Finkler, *Experiencing the New Genetics: Family and Kinship on the Medical Frontier* (Philadelphia: University of Pennsylvania Press, 2000).

74 N. M. Hadler and S. Greenhalgh, "Labeling Woefulness: The Social Construction of Fibromyalgia," *Spine* 30 (2005): 1–4.

75 L. I. Iezzoni and V. A. Freedman, "Turning the Disability Tide: The Importance of Definitions," *JAMA* 299 (2008): 332–34.

Chapter Nine

1 J. T. Cohen, P. J. Neumann, and M. C. Weinstein, "Does Preventive Care Save Money? Health Economics and the Presidential Candidates," *N Engl J Med* 358 (2008): 661–63; E. Golberstein, J. Liang, A. Quiñones, and F. D. Wolinsky, "Does More Health Care Improve Health among Older Adults?," *Journal of Aging and Health* 19 (2007): 888–906.

2 R. Angelmar, S. Angelmar, and L. Kane, "Building Strong Condition Brands,"

Journal of Medical Marketing 7 (2007): 341–51; M. Mitka, "Direct-to-Consumer Advertising of Medical Devices under Scrutiny," JAMA 300 (2008): 1985–86.

3 D. J. Rothman, "Academic Medical Centers and Financial Conflicts of Interest," JAMA 299 (2008): 695–97.

4 B. L. Martin, R. A. Deyo, S. K. Mirza, J. A. Turner, B. A. Comstock, W. Hollingworth, and S. D. Sullivan, "Expenditures and Health Status among Adults with Back and Neck Problems," JAMA 299 (2008): 656–64.

5 N. M. Hadler, The Last Well Person: How to Stay Well Despite the Health Care System (Montreal: McGill-Queens University Press, 2004); N. M. Hadler, Worried Sick: A Prescription for Health in an Overtreated America (Chapel Hill: University of North Carolina Press, 2008).

6 R. Bayer, L. O. Gostin, B. Jennings, and B. Steinbock, eds., Public Health Ethics: Theory, Policy, and Practice (Oxford: Oxford University Press, 2007).

7 D. Kuh and Y. Ben-Shlomo, eds., A Life Course Approach to Chronic Disease Epidemiology (Oxford: Oxford University Press, 1997).

8 N. M. Hadler, "A Ripe Old Age," Archives of Internal Medicine 163 (2003): 1261–62.

9 M. E. Williams and N. M. Hadler, "The Illness as the Focus of Geriatric Medicine," N Engl J Med 308 (1983): 1357–60.

10 M. Marmot, The Status Syndrome: How Social Standing Affects Our Health and Longevity (New York: Henry Holt, 2004).

11 I. Kawachi and L. F. Berkman, eds., Neighborhoods and Health (Oxford: Oxford University Press, 2003); M. Winkleby, C. Cubbin, and D. Ahn, "Low Individual Socioeconomic Status, Neighborhood Socioeconomic Status and Adult Mortality," American Journal of Public Health 96 (2006): 2145–53.

12 I. Kawachi, B. P. Kennedy, and R. G. Wilkinson, eds., The Society and Population Health Reader, vol. 1, Income Inequality and Health (New York: The New Press, 1999); N. M. Hadler, "Rheumatology and the Health of the Workforce," Arthritis Rheum 44 (2001): 1971–74.

13 J.-P. Michel, J. L. Newton, and T. B. L. Kirkwood, "Medical Challenges of Improving the Quality of a Longer Life," JAMA 299 (2008): 688–90.

14 N. Gilbert, Transformation of the Welfare State: The Silent Surrender of Public Responsibility (Oxford: Oxford University Press, 2004).

15 S. W. Glickman, F.-S. Ou, E. R. DeLong, M. T. Roe, B. L. Lytle, J. Mulgund, J. S. Rumsfeld, W. B. Gibler, E. M. Ohman, K. A. Schulman, and E. D. Peterson, "Pay for Performance, Quality of Care and Outcomes in Acute Myocardial Infarction," JAMA 297 (2007): 2373–80.

16 Hadler, The Last Well Person; Hadler, Worried Sick.

17 E. von Elm, D. G. Altman, M. Egger, S. J. Pocock, P. C. Gøtzsche, and J. P. Vandenbroucke, "Strengthening the Reporting of Observational Studies in Epidemiology (STROBE) Statement: Guidelines for Reporting Observational Studies," Ann Intern Med 147 (2007): 573–77.

18 N. Freemantle, "Observational Evidence for Determining Drug Safety Is No Substitute for Evidence from Randomised Controlled Trials," BMJ 336 (2008): 627–28.

19 Hadler, *Worried Sick*, pp. 244–48.

20 P. A. Halvorsen, R. Selmer, and I. S. Kristiansen, "Different Ways to Describe the Benefits of Risk-Reducing Treatments," *Ann Intern Med* 146 (2007): 848–56.

21 P. Slovic, M. Finucane, E. Peters, and D. G. MacGregor, "Risk as Analysis and Risk as Feelings: Some Thoughts about Affect, Reason, Risk, and Rationality," *Risk Analysis* 24, no. 2 (2004): 1–12.

22 G. Rose, *The Strategy of Preventive Medicine* (Oxford: Oxford University Press, 1992).

23 D. Hunter, "First, Gather the Data," *N Engl J Med* 354 (2006): 329–31.

24 S. W. Smith, "Sidelining Safety—The FDA's Inadequate Response to the IOM," *N Engl J Med* 357 (2007): 960–63; B. M. Psaty and R. A. Charo, "FDA Responds to Institute of Medicine Drug Safety Recommendations—In Part," *JAMA* 297 (2007): 1917–20.

25 T. H. Lee, "'Me-too' Products—Friend or Foe?," *N Engl J Med* 350 (2004): 211–12.

26 L. A. Cobb, G. I. Thomas, D. H. Dillard, and others, "An Evaluation of Internal-Mammary Ligation by a Double-Blind Technique," *N Engl J Med* 260 (1959): 1115–18.

27 Ibid.

28 J. B. Staal, R. de Bie, H. C. W. de Vet, J. Hildebrandt, and P. Nelemans, "Injection Therapy for Subacute and Chronic Low-Back Pain" (review), Cochrane Database of Systematic Reviews (2008), issue 3, art. no. CD001824, DOI: 10.1002/14651858. CD001824.pub3.

29 J. B. Moseley, K. O'Malley, N. J. Petersen, and others, "A Controlled Trial of Arthroscopic Surgery for Osteoarthritis of the Knee," *N Engl J Med* 347 (2002): 81–88.

30 F. G. Miller, "Sham Surgery: An Ethical Analysis," *American Journal of Bioethics* 3, no. 4 (2003): 41–48.

31 Hadler, *Worried Sick*, pp. 15–32.

32 Ibid.

33 S. H. Ehringhaus, J. S. Weissman, J. L. Sears, S. D. Goold, S. Feibelmann, and E. G. Campbell, "Responses of Medical Schools to Institutional Conflicts of Interest," *JAMA* 299 (2008): 665–71.

34 N. M. Hadler and the Ethics Forum, "Would Physician Disclosure of All Industry Gifts Solve the Conflict-of-Interest Problem? Negative Constructive," *American Medical News*, January 7, 2008.

35 N. M. Hadler and D. B. Gillings, "On the Design of the Phase III Drug Trial," *Arthritis Rheum* 26 (1983): 1354–61.

36 N. M. Hadler, "The Health Assurance, Disease Insurance Plan: Harnessing Reason to the Benefits of Employees," *Journal of Occupational and Environmental Medicine* 47 (2005): 655–57.

37 R. S. Braithwaite, M. S. Roberts, and A. C. Justice, "Incorporating Quality of Evidence into Decision Analytic Modeling," *Ann Intern Med* 146 (2007): 133–41.

38 R. L. Wears and M. Berg, "Computer Technology and Clinical Work: Still Waiting for Godot," *JAMA* 293 (2005): 1261–63.

39 R. A. McNutt, "Shared Medical Decision Making: Problems, Process, Progress," *JAMA* 292 (2004): 2516–18.

40 L. E. Boulware, S. Marinopoulos, K. A. Phillips, and others, "Systematic Review: The Value of the Periodic Health Evaluation," *Ann Intern Med* 146 (2007): 289–300.

41 Hadler, *Worried Sick.*

42 R. Maharaj, "Adding Cost to NNT: COPE Statistic," ACP *Journal Club* 148 (2008): A-8.

43 H.-G. Gadamer, *The Enigma of Health: The Art of Healing in a Scientific Age*, trans. J. Gaiger and N. Walker (Stanford: Stanford University Press, 1996), p. 107.

44 R. Buchbinder, D. P. Gross, E. L. Werner, and J. A. Hayden, "Understanding the Characteristics of Effective Mass Media Campaigns for Back Pain and Methodological Challenges in Evaluating Their Effects," *Spine* 33 (2008): 4–80.

ABOUT THE AUTHOR

NORTIN M. HADLER, M.D., M.A.C.P., F.A.C.R., F.A.C.O.E.M. (A.B. Yale University, M.D. Harvard Medical School), trained at the Massachusetts General Hospital, the National Institutes of Health in Bethesda, Maryland, and the Clinical Research Centre in London. He joined the faculty of the University of North Carolina in 1973 and was promoted to professor of medicine and microbiology/immunology in 1985. He serves as attending rheumatologist at the University of North Carolina Hospitals.

For thirty years, Dr. Hadler has been a student of the "illness of work incapacity"; over 200 scientific papers and thirteen books bear witness to this interest. He has lectured widely, garnered multiple awards, and served lengthy visiting professorships in England, France, Israel, and Japan. He has been elected to membership in the American Society for Clinical Investigation and the National Academy of Social Insurance. He is a student of the approach taken by many nations to the challenges of applying disability and compensation insurance schemes to such predicaments as back pain and arm pain in the workplace. He has dissected the fashion in which medicine turns disputative and thereby iatrogenic in the process of disability determination, whether for back or arm pain or for a more global illness narrative such as is labeled "fibromyalgia." He is widely regarded for his critical assessment of the limitations of certainty regarding medical and surgical management of the regional musculoskeletal disorders. Furthermore, he has applied his critical razor to much that is considered contemporary medicine at its finest.

The third edition of Dr. Hadler's monograph *Occupational Musculoskeletal Disorders* was published by Lippincott Williams & Wilkins in 2005 and provides a ready resource as to his thinking on all the regional musculoskeletal disorders. *The Last Well Person: How to Stay Well Despite the Health-Care System* was published by McGill-Queens University Press in 2004 and released in paperback in 2007. A French translation, *Le Dernier des Bien-Portants*, was published by Les Presses de l'Université Laval/Les Éditions de l'IQRC in 2008. It is a treatise on medicalization. A treatise on what Dr. Hadler calls Type II Medical Malpractice, *Worried Sick: A Prescription for Health in an Overtreated America*, was published by UNC Press in 2008. It was chosen by the Caravan Project (⟨www.caravanbooks.org⟩) for simultaneous release as an e-book, a large-print-format paperback, and an audio book.

INDEX

Disease-insurance account, 155, 156–60
Distress. *See* Psychological distress
Doctor-patient relationship, uncertainty in, 25
Dogmatist school of medicine, 55, 56
Drugs. *See* Prescription drugs

Ecological sampling, 13–14, 15
Education: back-care, 122, 128; back pain and, *18*
Edwin Smith Papyrus, 7
Effectiveness: definition of, 144; ergonomics on, 107; of health-care system, 144–47; number needed to treat and, 146, 156–57
Efficacy: definition of, 144; of health-care system, 144–47; randomized controlled trials testing for, 46, 144–47; of regional backache treatments, 48; of surgical devices, 148
Efficiency, ergonomics on, 107
Egypt, ancient, sciatica in, 6–7
Elizabethan era: poor laws in, 93; sciatica in, 7
Eminence-based medicine, 40, 73
Employment status, back pain and, *18*
Enablement fund, 155, 156, 159
Enablement state, 142–43
Engels, Friedrich, 95
Epidemics (Hippocrates), 73
Epidemiology: bias in, 13, 14; of cholera, 12; confounding in, 13, 14; descriptive, 12; life-course, 141, 160–61; role of, 12; roots of, 12; of scurvy, 12. *See also* Community epidemiology
Ergonomics, 107–9, 122
Ergonomics Working Group, 110–11
Erichsen, John Eric, 8–9
Ethics, 73, 92
Ethnicity. *See* Race/ethnicity
Evidence: for efficacy, 46, 144; level of, 46, 47

Evidence-based medicine, 47
Evidence-based treatment, of regional backache, 46–48
Examinations, independent medical, 125–27, 133–34
Exposure-based therapies, for posttraumatic stress disorder, 57

Facet joints, 43
Family Assistance Plan, 100
FDA. *See* Food and Drug Administration
Fear avoidance, 119
Fellow-servant doctrine, 95
Fibromyalgia: cerebral functional imaging of, 36; criteria for classification of, 31; definition of, 28; drugs for, 36; label of, 25–26, 31, 36; pathogenesis of, 25; psychological distress in, 31, 32; semiotics of, 31–33; social construction of, 25–26; verbal dimension of, 31. *See also* Chronic musculoskeletal pain
Fibrous annulus, 79
Financial interests. *See* Commercial interests
"Financial Ties Are Cited as Issue in Spine Study" (Abelson), 92
Finland: study on lifting tasks in, 110; trial on discectomy in, 85
"Fixed and stable," *102, 117,* 120–21, 125, 127
Flexeril (cyclobenzaprine hydrochloride), 31
Folk diagnosis, of posttraumatic stress disorder, 56–57
Folk remedies, for posttraumatic stress disorder, 57
Food, Drug, and Cosmetic Act (1938), 74, 77
Food and Drug Administration (FDA): calculating number needed to treat from data of, 156; on fibromyalgia, 36; on new drugs, 150; on surgical

Illness-disease paradigm, 28, 29, 39, 52, 56, 129, 134
Imaging of spine, 40–45, 42–43; cost of, 44; futility of, 41, 44–45; patient satisfaction and, 44
IME. *See* Independent medical examinations
Imhotep, 6–7
Impairment-based disability determination, 129–37; Kafka on, 130–31; limitations of, 129; in Prussia, 21, 129–31; in United States, 131–37
Income maintenance, 99, 100, 101
Income tax, negative, 100, 101
Independent medical examinations (IMEs), 125–27, 133–34
Industrial Age: human cost of, 95; poor laws in, 94–95; Railway Spine in, 8–9, 34; workers' compensation in, 9–10, 96–97, 102
Inferior articular process, 43
Injection, intradiscal, 77–81
Injury: from defective devices, 75–76, 147–48; workplace, in Industrial Age, 95. *See also* Regional back injury
Insoles, trials on, 48
Institute for Workers' Health and Safety, 49
Institute of Medicine, 57, 147
Institute of Occupational Health (Finland), 110
Insurance: social, 103, 136–37; workers purchasing, 96. *See also* Health insurance
Intervertebral disc. *See* Disc
Interview, clinical, 157–58
Intradiscal electrothermal annuloplasty and nucleotomy (IDET), 80–81, 149
Intradiscal injection, 77–81
Islam, on charity, 93

Jenner, Edward, 56

Job dissatisfaction. *See* Work dissatisfaction
Johnson, Lyndon B., 100
Johnson & Johnson, 91
Joint Commission on Accreditation of Healthcare Organizations, 120
Judges. *See* Administrative law judges

Kafka, Franz, 130–31, 154
Kantian welfare state, 140
Kefauver-Harris Amendment (1962), 77
Kennedy, John F., 72–73, 87
"Keyhole" laminectomy, 83
King, Martin Luther, Jr., 101
Kosher meat, 6n
Krankenkassen, 96

Labeling, of fibromyalgia, 25–26, 31, 36
Lamina, *43*, 82–83
Laminectomy, *43*, 82–83; history of, 82; "keyhole," 83; procedure of, 83; regional variation in, 84
Lasègue, Charles, 7
Lasègue's Sign, 7
Lassalle, Ferdinand, 9, 95
Level of evidence, 46, 47
Liberty Mutual, 107
Life Chiropractic College, 66
Life-course epidemiology, 141, 160–61
Life expectancy, 141
Life University, 66
Lifting tasks, 106, 110
Limpieza (cleansing), 57, 59
Lind, James, 12
Lister, Joseph, 56
Lloyd George, David, 95, 97
Loisel, P., 122
London, Jack, 9, 94
London Labour and the London Poor (Mayhew), 94–95
Longitudinal studies, 19, 22
Love, Grafton, 83

Nachemson, Alf, 85
Napropaths, 66
National Business Group on Health, 152
National Center for Health Statistics, 16
National Health Interview Survey (NHIS), 16–19, *18*, 20
National Institute for Health and Clinical Excellence (NICE), 51
National Institute of Occupational Safety and Health (NIOSH), 108, 109
National Institutes of Health (NIH), 150
National Insurance Administration (Norway), 121, 122
National Population Health Survey (NPHS), 21
Naturopaths, 66
Negative income tax, 100, 101
Nemiah, John C., 10
Nerve: pinched, 1; sciatic, 6–7, 6n, 79, 127
Nerve root compression, 132
Netherlands: trial on discectomy in, 85; workers' compensation in, 97, 115
Neuroasthenia, Railway Spine as, 9
Neuropaths, 66
Neurophysiology, of chronic musculoskeletal pain, 34–36
New drug application (NDA), 150–52, 159
New England Journal of Medicine, 1
News (AMA), 89
New York Times, 88–89, 90, 92
New Zealand: guidelines for backache treatment in, 49; workers' compensation in, 97
NIH. *See* National Institutes of Health
NIOSH. *See* National Institute of Occupational Safety and Health
Nixon, Richard, 100
NNT. *See* Number needed to treat
Nonsteroidal anti-inflammatory drugs, trials on, 48
North American Spine Society, 51

North Carolina Back Pain Project, 70
Norway: disability-insurance scheme in, 121–22; trial on discectomy in, 85; trial on spinal fusion in, 88
Nucleotome, 81, 82
Nucleotomy. *See* Intradiscal electrothermal annuloplasty and nucleotomy
Nucleus pulposus (NP), *78, 79*; injection of, 77–81; posterolateral herniation of, 79; removal of, 81–86
Number needed to treat (NNT), 146, 156–57, 159, 160

Observational studies, 144
Occupational medicine, 108
Occupational neurosis, 10, 104
Occupational Safety and Health Act (1970), 108
Occupational Safety and Health Administration (OSHA), 108
Office of Economic Opportunity, 101
Old Age and Disability Insurance (1889), 96
Old Testament, 6, 93
Omnibus Budget Reconciliation Act (1989), 50
Onik, Gary, 81–82
Ontario Workplace Safety and Insurance Board, 115
Opioid analgesia, 123–24, 127
Oratec, 80, 81
Organized labor. *See* Trade unions
Orthopaedic medicine, 68–70
Orwell, George, 9, 94
Osteopathy, 65–66, 68–70
Osteophytes, 40

Paget, Sir James, 65
Pain. *See specific types of pain*
Pain clinics, 127–28
Paine, Thomas, 101
Pain generator, 76, 83, 84, 86, 90
Painkillers, 123–24

State-based health-care system, 155, 156

Statins, 145

Still, Andrew Taylor, 64–65

Straight chiropractic, 66–67, 68

Strict test, 131–32

Subluxations, 67, 68

Superior articular process, 43

Supplemental Security Income (SSI), 103, 133–35, 137, 162

Surgeons: ancient punishments for, 72; as heroes, 74; innovations by, 74. See also Spine surgeons

Surgery: history of, 72; improvement in techniques of, 74. See also Spine surgery

Surgical devices, 147–50; approval of, 75, 76, 87, 147–48; classification of, 74; definition of, 74, 75; for disc arthroplasty, 90–92; for discectomy, 82; for intradiscal injection, 80–81; laissez-faire attitude toward, 74; for spinal fusion, 87, 88–90; tort immunity for defective, 75–76, 147–48; trials on, 148–50; whistle-blower suits on, 90

Surrogate complaint, 54, 109–12, 123

Surveys: community, 15–16, 38–39, 39, 114–15; methodology of, 16; postal, 19, 22, 23–25, 24

Susto, 56–57

Sweden: trial on spinal fusion in, 87–88; whiplash-associated disorders in, 57

Swedish Lumbar Spine Study Group, 87–88

Switzerland, workers' compensation in, 97

Sydenham, Thomas, 28, 29, 39, 40, 56, 129

Synthes Spine, Inc., 91, 92

Tait, Raymond, 125

Telegraphist's wrist, 10, 104

Tender points, 31

Tenet Healthcare, 89

Texas Back Institute, 89, 91, 92

Tichauer, Erwin, 107

TNF-alpha inhibitors, 159–60

Tobin, James, 101

Tort immunity, 76, 104

Tort systems: on injury from defective device, 75–76, 147–48; whiplash-associated disorders and, 57–58; workers' compensation schemes and, 104

Trade unions, 95–96, 107, 108

Traumatic neurosis: Railway Spine as, 9; workers' injuries as, 10, 104

Treatment: aggressive, 26–27, 73–74; conservative, 26, 73–74; vs. treatment act, 62. See also Modality

Treatment act: of acupuncturist, 60, 62; becoming patient in, 53; clinical interview as part of, 157; definition of, 62; maladaptive illness behaviors and, 30; modality in, 48, 62; spinal manipulation as part of, 70–71; vs. treatment, 62

Trial, The (Kafka), 130, 131

Trials. See Randomized controlled trials; Sham-controlled trials

Type II Medical Malpractice, 143, 154

Tzedakah (charity), 93

Uncertainty, in doctor-patient relationship, 25

Union movement, 95–96, 104, 107, 108

U.S. Preventive Services Task Force, 146

University of California College, 65

University of Cincinnati, 108

University of Michigan, 107, 108

University of North Carolina, 125

University of North Carolina Trial of Spinal Manipulation, 69, 69–70

Utilitarian welfare state, 140

Vegetative life, 33

Verbrugge, Lois, 15